This book is dedicated to my endlessly supportive family; my wife, Leah; and our two boys, Jake and Zach. They are the reasons I leave for work so early in the morning and come home every night. Thank you for all of your support.

Contents

Preface

"TINSTAAFEL."

It was written in gritty white chalk on the side blackboard of my seventh grade science classroom on the very first day. As we listened to Mr. Weaver introduce himself and tell us what we could expect to learn that year, all of us kept glancing over at the word on the board. Nobody knew what it meant. TINSTAAFEL. What could it be? Was it something we were already supposed to know? A test of some kind? Curiosity burned. Finally, someone was brave enough to ask what it meant. With a smile that told us he'd been waiting for that question, Mr. Weaver replied, "If there is anything you remember from me or my class, it should be this word. It stands for 'There Is No Such Thing As a Free Lunch.'" TINSTAAFEL. This was a critical lesson for middle schoolers just starting to make their way into adulthood, introduced and made memorable by initially saying nothing at all about it. Mr. Weaver taught me a lot, and not just about science. He was a wonderful teacher, able to keep seventh graders engaged by infusing science class with fun and stories. But what I carry with me is TINSTAAFEL: In this life, if you want something you need to work for it. His words, and his gift for teaching, stuck with me.

For years I've been teaching advanced anatomical and physiological concepts to all levels of students, from those who have just started their careers to those who have been in the fitness industry for decades. It has always been my goal to focus and shape these concepts so that everyone can understand them without compromising the facts. All too often when simplifying a concept, instructors either patronize the students and talk down to them, or speak so broadly that they skip over the important points of a concept to avoid overwhelming them. I believe that a good teacher can teach everyone the same information and skills, lifting up those who may not have as many years of experience to the level of those more knowledgeable, while simultaneously introducing concepts generally reserved for the more advanced student. But teaching just the facts can be dull. How many of us have looked forward to a lecture by a well regarded instructor who is a true expert in the field, only to be reminded that expertise does not guarantee good teaching skills? The instructor turns out to be dull and droning, lulling the audience into a trance. The information is there, but teaching is so much more than knowledge: A true teacher needs the ability to connect and entertain.

The goal is to combine this transfer of knowledge—challenging the students without patronizing them—with the kind of engaging rhetoric that made Mr. Weaver's class so memorable. My dear friend Nora has called this teaching style "infotainment." It's the perfect mixture of 30 percent information, 10 percent passion, 10 percent storytelling, and 50 percent fearlessness in making a fool of oneself. The ability to get the information across in a way that the students will understand—making it not only digestible but fun—requires taking risks and opening up with a vulnerability that allows the students to connect with you on a personal level and to be willing to take risks themselves. It isn't easy, and it has taken me a long time to develop my teaching style to be able to do just that.

I had just finished lecturing at an international fitness convention when a woman approached me and said two important things. First, she explained how much she had learned in my course titled "Anatomy in Three Dimensions: Common Spinal Conditions." She mentioned that my teaching style made it easy to understand the content without being patronizing or dumbing it down, and that she had learned more in this class than perhaps in any other spinal course. I was touched that she had taken the time to express how much she had gotten out of the class, and gratified to hear that my efforts to provide information in a useful way had been successful. I have heard this from many students since I started teaching, but every time it is a reminder of how hard I have worked to truly connect with my students, and it reinvigorates me to keep working on new and different ways to reach those who take my courses.

There is a danger, though, in putting too much stock in the fun and not enough emphasis on the learning. "Radar," as I called my high school history teacher because he looked so much like the actor Gary Burghoff, who played Radar O'Reilly in *M.A.S.H.*, kept us in stitches. His classes were great fun, almost too much so. After the first quarter of the year, everyone was failing. It seems we thought of his class as a show, not a course. We got so caught up in his stories and jokes that we didn't bother learning the material. Radar gave us a talking-to that I will never forget. He told us that if everyone, and he meant everyone, didn't get an A in the next quarter, we would all fail. We figured out how to learn from him and have fun at the same time. This taught me the value of substance and style being equal. You can't have one overpower the other, or one will be drowned out.

I have had some wonderful teachers in my life, some who have had lasting effects on me and have shaped the person, and instructor, I am today. My mom, Gabrielle, got me into the fitness game and taught me how to see the body differently from everyone else, and how to trust my intuition. My dad, Bob, taught me the art of "talking story": how to tell stories that illustrate your point and draw people in. My stepfather, Alex, showed me patience and taught me to listen before responding and acting. Dr. Mike Jones taught me medical exercise and led me down the path to what I do today. My college professors instilled the discipline to keep going even when the journey's end seemed far away. My friend, mentor, and twin brain, Nora St. John, saw me as an equal, and she continues to challenge me and lift me up to be an even better teacher and instructor. And finally, my wife, Leah, and our children, Jake and Zach, have taught me to believe in myself by doing so themselves. They light the way back home.

I stand on the shoulders of giants. I am not a self-made man. Who I am today is the culmination of all the teachers from whom I have learned, as well as all the students I have taught. In every class I take and teach, I learn something that shapes me, and for that I am so fortunate and incredibly grateful. I am privileged to be able to call myself a teacher, and I can only hope that I leave a strong impression on my students that sticks with them as they travel on their journeys. It would be my greatest honor to have them remember me not just as an expert in my field but as a wonderful teacher who helped them grow and who gave them a lesson that has served them as well as TINSTAAFEL has served me.

I hope this teaching style for which I have worked so hard comes through in each chapter of this book. It is filled with a lot of facts and anatomy, but presented in a way that makes it relatable and enjoyable to read. Whether you are a seasoned fitness enthusiast or someone who knows nothing about the body and claims to have an allergic reaction to exercise, I hope you will get something out of this book. You will ultimately know exactly what is going on in your lower back and how to manage it with exercise.

Oh, and remember the woman who spoke to me after my class? Remember how I wrote that she told me two things? The second was actually a question. She asked, "Have you ever thought of writing a book?"

Acknowledgments

I am grateful to have such wonderful support and help in creating this book. I'd like to say "Mahalo Nui Loa" to:

Nora St. John and Balanced Body for welcoming me in like family and supporting my creative ideas and endeavors. You gave me a spotlight to shine and I hope to always live up to your high standards.

Megan Wentland, PhD, editor script doctor, and wordsmith extraordinaire. It's critical to have someone who understands your voice and can help craft it from the spoken word to the written page.

And finally to every client and student I have worked with in the past 25 or more years. While school and academics gave me a foundation, it's the hands-on experience that made me the practitioner I am today.

Introduction

In the age of the Internet, we have become a society that believes we can self-diagnose with a few clicks and self-heal by reading a book or a website. I understand the temptation—who wants to go to the time and expense of seeing a doctor when a quick stop at the bookstore holds the answer? Here's the thing: This is not that kind of book. It's a help, a guide, or a way forward *after* you have consulted with a doctor. There are so many parts of your body that connect to your spine that to suggest otherwise would be irresponsible, because you can do real damage to your long-term health if you try to self-diagnose or self-treat. This book is not to be used in place of medical treatment. If you are in pain, the first thing you need to do is make an appointment with your doctor and get a diagnosis. In the meantime, you are welcome to read this book to help you understand your potential diagnosis and see what your treatment may entail, because my goal is to inform and educate you about your medical condition and guide you toward exercises that will help manage your specific condition. Once you have a diagnosis and a treatment plan, you can use the guides and exercises in this book to augment and maintain your health going forward.

How To Use This Book

"Move Better, Stand Taller, and Exercise Pain Free."

This is the mission statement of my exercise studio and a motto that I use as the basis of programing with every client. Over the years I have noticed that pleasure and pain are opposite sides of the same coin, and both are very powerful motivators. In fact, in his essay "Beyond the Pleasure Principle," Dr. Sigmund Freud noted how people will often go to great lengths to avoid pain, even if it is temporary and mild. While Dr. Freud was talking primarily about psychological issues, I've seen this concept mirrored in my practice when clients are dealing with physical pain. I'd be willing to bet that pain is what led you to pick up this book. You're probably at the point where you've had enough and are ready to take control of your back pain rather than letting it have control over you. Good for you!

I know it's hard to face pain. For years, I lived every day with debilitating back pain that was caused by obesity as a child and young adult. At one point I weighed over 400 pounds (181 kg). This crushing weight damaged some portions of my spine, leaving me in a great deal of pain. Even after I lost the weight I still had daily pain, because the damage was already done and does not magically undo itself. I consulted many physicians and physical therapists looking for a quick treatment or a medicine that would help, but no one had the answer I was looking for. Eventually I realized that I was looking for someone else to "fix" me. I wanted them to do the work and perform the miracle, while I reaped the benefits. It doesn't work that way. I had to use the knowledge I had and work to fix myself.

I've spent most of my career working with clients in pain. As a personal trainer specializing in medical exercise, I have the ability to help other people manage their medical conditions with exercise. I can encourage them to work hard toward pain relief. But I couldn't seem to help myself until I came to this realization. What changed? A number of things changed, but first was my attitude. I took a hard look at myself and asked, "How hard have you really been trying?" I was forced to recognize that I hadn't been trying nearly as hard as I could or should have been. I reminded myself of what I have often told clients: Accomplishing anything comes down to six words: "How bad do you want it?" If you want to see a change, you've got to really want it, and then do whatever it takes to make it happen.

So I made changes. I worked harder—a lot harder. I became stronger, and soon the pain lessened. Before long, it was gone. Initially, I was pain-free for only a few days at a time, but eventually there were longer and longer stretches in which I wasn't in constant pain and discomfort. Sure, from time to time it returned, but never as bad as it had been. When it did return, I knew that I needed to resume the exercises that had worked so well the first time, and each time I was able to recover quickly. Ultimately, I saw that when I put in the effort, my relapses were less intense, less frequent, and shorter in duration. That's my hope for you as well.

Within the pages of this book you will find a guide to managing your low back pain (LBP). You won't find a secret or a speedy fix: The secret, as I explained above, is your choice to commit to your wellness. My goal is to empower you with the exercises and skills it takes for you to take control of your LBP, to help you to take back your life and not let pain prevent you from doing the activities that make up your life. But in the end, you have to choose to do the exercises. Just buying the book won't get you anywhere. You have the power to make a change, but you have to put in the time and effort.

This book is divided into three parts: The Spinal Unit, Exercises, and Common Conditions. Part I The Spinal Unit is very important. The first chapter, Anatomy of the Spine, provides you with a foundation to understand everything else that follows. Without understanding the anatomy of the spine, you will have a very difficult time understanding your specific spinal condition and may end up frustrated. Don't be tempted to skip it: Learning the anatomy helps set the table for the meal you are about to eat. This part also includes chapter 2 Spinal Stability Training, which explains how to build and increase spinal stability, and chapter 3 Assess Yourself, which teaches you how to gauge pain and assess your posture.

Part II Exercises describes all of the exercises related to the lower back. They are grouped together by exercise type—chapter 4 covers supine and prone exercises; chapter 5 covers quadruped, seated, and standing exercises;

and chapter 6 covers mobility and flexibility exercises. It is critical to note that not all of these exercises are appropriate for all spinal conditions. In fact, some of them are contraindicated for certain conditions. That's why it is important to understand the anatomy and pathology of your specific condition. If you jump into the exercises without knowing which exercises are best for you, you will be wasting your time at best and run the risk of seriously injuring yourself at worst. My suggestion is to skim through this section to learn how the types of exercises build upon each other, but don't linger or get too fixed on any particular series. Instead, return to this section once you have read the chapter relating to your specific condition. The exercises will make much more sense once you understand how they'll help you work towards wellness.

Part III Common Conditions brings everything together. This part includes chapters on each specific spinal condition, the goals and contraindications for each, and then a specific exercise program for you to follow for each condition. You don't need to read about all the conditions, unless you're interested in continuing to learn more about the physiology and different pathologies of the back. The aim is for you to simply turn to the chapter that corresponds to your condition and read that one. You will see that each workout is divided into a schedule of months. Plan to complete the workout schedules starting at the first month and progressing through as you get stronger.

How To Read This Book

Here is how I think the book is best read: Start with part I to learn about spinal anatomy, spinal stability, and how to assess your posture and gauge your pain. Then just skim—or even skip—part II for right now, and go right to your specific spinal condition in part III and read that chapter—maybe even read it twice. When you get to the exercise plan for your condition, return to part II to find and highlight or mark the specific exercises that you are going to be doing for the first month and learn those. For additional information and selected videos explaining some of the foundational and more difficult exercises, you can visit www.backexercisebook.com. When you have completed the first month and are ready to progress to the second month, return to part II to learn the new exercises, and continue as you go forward each month.

This is the most efficient way to use the book and make the most of it. As you are doing the exercises, ideally you will begin to feel stronger and progressively in less discomfort. Many clients begin to feel better in a matter of weeks, but it's important to continue doing the exercises through the full cycle even if you are feeling better and have no pain. You will be getting stronger, but the process won't be complete for some time. Think chess, not checkers—you're playing the long game. You want to be strong for the long haul, not just for the short term. This program is designed help you do that, if you trust the plan.

In the following pages, I will guide you toward a life of increased activity, more pain-free days, and a greater quality of life. As you turn the next page, you are making the choice to work toward your pain-free future.

PART I

The Spinal Unit

"I've hurt my back, what should I do?" This message was recently emailed to me from a client who was away from home and away from her go-to low back pain remedies, hoping that I had some insight on pain relief. I can't tell you how many times in my career I have received a variation of this question in an email or a phone call. How I wish that there were an easy, single-sentence answer I could have given her, something that would have solved her problem quickly and easily, but alas, there wasn't. Every person's back problem is unique, so there is no one treatment that will fit everyone. Granted, the anatomy is the same—we all have roughly the same body structure—but how we have used and abused that structure is where the complications arise. The only "fixes" are time, patience, and hard work. The first section of this book will help you begin.

Anatomy is first. Without a clear understanding of how the body fits together and functions, it will be impossible to really understand how and why the exercises will help. The anatomy information is the foundation on which everything else is built. Your individual diagnosis, or pathology, is what determines the course of your exercise choices: You will use it to design a program to stabilize and strengthen your back.

In the first chapter, you learn about spinal anatomy—the basic information needed to understand what has happened in your spine based on your diagnosis. The second chapter introduces you to the concept of spinal stabilization and why it's so important to help you strengthen your low back. Finally, in chapter three you perform a self-assessment to provide a baseline of your condition, so you know exactly where you're starting; it will give you some perspective against which to measure your progress.

These chapters are going to be the first steps in your journey to learning how to manage your low back pain. Each chapter will provide you with the necessary information to understand the *why* behind the chosen exercises in the later chapters. My goal is to give you the tools and guidance to take control of your pain and to manage it through the exercises prescribed later. Once you understand the information about your particular condition, then you will be able to make better choices in your daily life to keep your back pain at bay. By reading these chapters, you're taking charge of your pain and choosing to not allow it to dominate your life.

CHAPTER 1

Anatomy of the Spine

The human body is often likened to a machine. In fact, it is often called the perfect machine. Think about it. For what we ask this machine to do, it is as remarkably complex as it is resilient. However, like any machine, wear and tear can take its toll. Through not only athletic endeavors, but simply through daily activities, your body's joints are asked to perform thousands of similar movement repetitions. Whether you are a runner logging hard-pounding miles, or a tennis player breaking and charging on the court, or a golfer performing hundreds of swings in the same direction during each round (counting practice strokes), the effect it has on your ankles, knees, hip, shoulders, and especially spinal joints is enormous. The fact that these joints last as long as they do is remarkable.

But like most "machines," we too can break down over time. Dr. Ronald Hetzler, my Professor of Exercise Physiology, once remarked to our class that our bodies have a limited warranty of 70 years. While that is a bit simplistic, it's quite apropos. Our joints are made up of connective tissue, including tendons, ligaments, and cartilage, which do deteriorate—albeit very slowly—over time. Some people tend to break down more rapidly than others, due to their body's genetics or their activity level. We need to do everything we can to slow down this process and minimize the effects of Mother Nature.

The spine is the literal backbone of our machine, and is possibly the most complicated series of joints in the body. In this chapter we will delve into the spine, specifically the lumbar portion, discussing not only the musculature but also the other connective tissues that comprise this remarkable structure.

I understand that not everyone wants to dive deep into the anatomy, physiology, and kinesiology of the spine. "Just tell me what to do and let me do it" is something I hear way too often. But let me offer you something to think about. The exercises that I suggest later in this book are very important for building up your core strength and stability, and understanding the "why" behind each exercise is incredibly important as well. If you understand why you are doing the exercises, then you are more likely to actually do the exercises and perform them properly. I know I tend to drive my personal training staff a bit crazy with the "why." I am infamous for walking up behind them while they are training a client and whispering, "Why?" When they hear this, they know that I want them to justify why they chose that particular exercise for that particular client. Any exercise you do has to have a reason, otherwise you're just wasting time and money.

So, for those of you who want to truly understand why you are doing these exercises, then please read on. For those who are more impatient, skip forward to the chapters on your specific pathology or injury and the corresponding exercises. But remember that these chapters are waiting for you when you are ready. Okay, let's begin.

Spinal Anatomy

First, let's discuss the importance of your spine. What does it do and why do you need it? The spine is critical for efficient movement of the body. It helps to integrate movements between the torso, pelvis, and shoulder girdle. Without a healthy, free-moving spine, the body is very limited as to what it can do. Throwing a ball or swinging a bat performed with arms only—without the use of the entire body—would be powerless. Believe it or not, most movements you do involve the entire body. Whether it is running for a bus, picking up a child, putting the laundry in the dryer, or unloading the dishwasher, you are using your entire body. A healthy, functioning spine is critical for all of these movements.

Another important feature of the spine is protection for our spinal column and nervous system. The bones of the spine enclose our spinal column, providing its own suit of armor and protecting it from damage. This also gives structure to our nervous system; our nerve endings exit the spine to each muscle and organ in the body. This structure creates a network mainframe from which all the wires (nerves) branch outward.

The Bones

The spine is made up of five distinct sections (see figure 1.1). Starting at the top and moving downward, we have the cervical spine comprised of seven bones, the thoracic spine comprised of twelve bones, the lumbar spine comprised of five bones, the sacrum made up of five fused bones, and finally the coccyx comprised of three to five small bones. Each section has a specific structure designed for its function, and each region has a curve unto itself. The cervical region curves inward (lordosis), the thoracic region curves outward (kyphosis), the lumbar curves back inward (lordosis), and the sacrum curves outward. These curves allow the spine to withstand stress and absorb forces.

Cervical Spine

The cervical region (the neck) is made up of the smallest vertebra and is designed for the largest range of motion. Move your head and neck around and you will see what I mean. Rotating it, tilting it forward and back, and side to side, you will see that you can move the neck in many different directions. Unlike some animals with eyes on the sides of their heads, we have our eyes on one side only. This gives us great depth perception but limits our field of vision. The ability to turn our

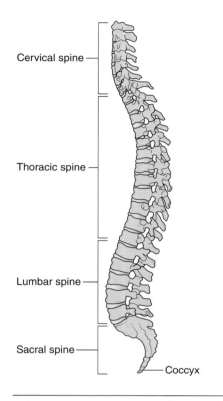

FIGURE 1.1   Five sections of the spine: cervical, thoracic, lumbar, sacrum, and coccyx.

necks and see up to 270 degrees around our bodies aided our ancestors in protection from enemies and predators as well as in hunting and scouting. It's this flexibility that gives us great advantages in vision but also creates an area of inherent weakness; a lot of injuries in the cervical region are due to arthritis, muscle strains, and fractures. These vertebrae are relatively small compared to their counterparts further down the spine, which is evident when looking at the "body," or front portion, of the vertebra. This is the round portion in the front of the vertebra that bears the weight of everything above it. Because it is near the top of the spinal column, it doesn't have as much weight to support as the areas below it. You can also see it in the articular surfaces, the posterior sections where the bones glide on each other and allow for muscle attachment, which are smaller and appear more delicate. Their shape and size allows the cervical region of the spine to have the greatest amount of movement.

Thoracic Spine

The vertebrae of the thoracic spine comprise the upper back. The vertebrae change as they travel down your spine. The front portion (body) of the vertebra get larger as they are required to support increasing weight. The spinous process (the part of the bone sticking out on the back) eventually begins to point at a downward angle rather than straight out. This, combined with the direction of the articular (mating) surfaces, allows for flexion, side-to-side movement, and limited extension, but the important thing to note is that it also allows a greater amount of rotation. In fact, most of the rotation that occurs in the trunk comes from the thoracic spine and not from the lumbar region (the waist).

Lumbar Spine

Traveling further down the spine, we come to the lumbar region. We cover this area in great detail because the low back is one of the most often injured areas of the body.

The lumbar spine contains the largest vertebrae in the spine, which makes sense because it carries the most weight and contributes greatly to the strength and stability of the entire body. Stability is incredibly important in this region. While the lumbar spine has great flexion, extension, and side-to-side movement, it does not allow for much rotation. In fact, each lumbar spinal segment rotates only one or two degrees. So, from your waist you only rotate 5 to 10 degrees total. That's not very much. The thoracic spine does the lion's share of trunk rotation. This thoracic rotation along with hip rotation makes you appear to be twisting at the waist, but the motion is really happening above and below your lumbar area. So, when you swing that golf club or tennis racket, you should focus on turning through the hips and shoulders and not at the waist. Forcing too much rotation from the lumbar spine will ultimately result in injury and pain.

Low Back Pain: Did You Know?

Here are a few facts about low back pain:

- Low back pain is the leading cause of disability worldwide.[1]
- Low back pain accounts for 264 million days of missed work annually.[2]
- It is estimated that nearly 80 percent of all people will suffer from low back pain at some time in their lives.[3]
- The cost of low back pain to our health care system is over $50 billion annually. If you factor in missed work and lost wages, that number climbs to over $100 billion dollars.[4]

Sacrum

The sacrum is located below your lumbar spine and is made up of five fused vertebrae. It is concave (kyphosis) in nature and serves as a connection between the spine and the pelvis (hip bones). The point at which the sacrum meets the pelvis is called your sacroiliac joint (SI joint) and it is an area where we occasionally see dysfunction. While the sacrum is seated between the two bones of the pelvis much like a keystone in an archway, sometimes the fit isn't as snug as it should be. Through use and abuse you may stretch out your sacroiliac (SI) ligaments leading to greater movement than desired. That, combined with too little or too much movement, can cause instability in the SI joints which in turn can produce dysfunction and pain. This could manifest itself as sciatic nerve pain in which feelings of numbness, tingling, or radiating pain down the leg can range from irritating to downright debilitating. This indicates muscular imbalance, whether it is an imbalance of one muscle being too tight and its corresponding muscle being too loose, or one muscle being too strong and its corresponding partner being too weak. Either scenario can cause the joint to get (and remain) out of alignment leading to faulty movement patterns which, if not addressed, can create lasting problems. For example, the piriformis muscle attaches from the hip to the sacrum. If one side gets too tight and the other is stretched beyond its normal length, the sacrum itself tilts to one side. If we view the entire spine as a chain, this shift in the sacrum can cause a shift all the way up the spine.

Coccyx

The coccyx is made up of three to five bones at the very bottom of your spine. Until we injure it, not much is mentioned about the coccyx (or tailbone). Injury is usually caused by a trauma, such as a fall or being struck by something. Unfortunately, a broken coccyx can lead to long-lasting pain and should be treated by a physician or physical therapist.

Intervertebral Disc

We cannot go any further without talking about another very important structure of our spinal column, the intervertebral disc. The disc is an amazing structure that can certainly be a pain.

The intervertebral disc is comprised of two areas (see figure 1.2). Like a jelly donut, with pastry on the outside and jelly on the inside, your disc also has external and internal portions. The outer portion is called the annulus fibrosis and is made up of fibrocartilage, which is really tough connective tissue. It has to be; think of how much motion your spine experiences on a daily basis, and multiply that by your age. Consider all the sporting events you've participated in and all the moving, twisting, and bending movements that you take for granted. The tough annulus fibrosis is

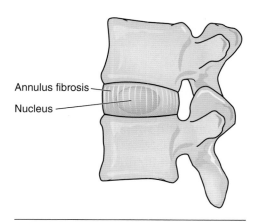

Annulus fibrosis

Nucleus

FIGURE 1.2   Intervertebral disc.

there to manage compressive forces, in other words, shock absorption. It is really good at its job—until it gets damaged. The annulus fibrosis is made up of seven to eighteen layers of fibrocartilage that are alternately arranged: One layer may be horizontal, the next diagonal, the next vertical, and so on, giving the disc strength and resiliency. If all the layers went in the same direction, the disc would be strong in handling certain forces but weak in others. Much like a tire on your car, each layer of steel belts embedded in the tire allow for it to move and flex as it goes around a turn, but at the same time be very strong. Similarly, the disc has to be able to withstand not only compressive forces for which it was designed, but also resist, support, and limit flexion and rotation. These layers of the annulus fibrosis allow it to distribute weight (forces) onto the vertebrae as well as protect the vertebral end plate which nourishes our discs.

The center of the disc is called the nucleus—the jelly in the donut so to speak. It is a gel-like structure comprised primarily of water that provides shock absorption. As forces are applied to your disc (donut), your nucleus moves depending on the nature and direction of the force. When a compressive force is applied to the disc, flattening out the jelly donut, the nucleus is evenly pushed out 360 degrees. If the force is applied only to the back of the disc (as if you are arching your back), the nucleus moves forward; if force is applied to the front of the disc (as if you are bending forward) then the nucleus is pushed backward. This becomes very important when we discuss disc herniations and bulges, because it is the nucleus that pushes its way through the annular fibers and causes trouble.

Muscles

We have talked about the bones, which are the framework for the spine, and now we must also discuss the muscles that align the spine. Think of these as the support mechanism that keeps the spine aligned, allowing it to move safely and return to its proper original position. Your body is comprised of two groups of muscles: mobilizers and stabilizers. The mobilizers are "mirror muscles"—the ones that you see in the mirror when you flex your muscles. These produce a lot of torque, meaning they are your power-generating muscles. With a predominance of type II muscle fibers, they build tension rapidly and are designed for strength over endurance, but tend to fatigue quickly and work better with higher amounts of resistance. Stabilizers, on the other hand, are located much deeper in the body. These are muscles you generally cannot see from the outside. Let's look at each group more closely.

Stabilizers of the Spine

The stabilizers are small muscles located close to the joint they stabilize. They primarily consist of slow-twitch muscle fibers (except for a select few), and do not provide a lot of power, but are built for endurance. Responsible for posture, they are often referred to as your "postural muscles," meaning they keep the joints in

Fast-Twitch Versus Slow-Twitch Muscles

Fast-twitch muscles fire quickly and are able to produce a lot of power, but the cost of producing this amount of power is that they fatigue easily. These muscles run out of energy (oxygen) quickly, so they are not meant for endurance, but for strength. They are the larger muscles that you can see in the mirror. The sprinter, Usain Bolt, for instance, has very large lower body muscles; being the "fastest man alive," you would expect that, but you wouldn't expect him to run a marathon. His muscles are built for quick bursts of speed and power.

Slow-twitch muscles are the endurance fibers. They don't produce nearly as much strength and power but can contract for a longer period of time and for a greater number of repetitions. Postural and stabilizing muscles fall into this category. There are also intermediate fibers that, depending on whether you train primarily for endurance or for power, will take on the characteristics of those fast- or slow-twitch fibers.

proper alignment allowing the joints to move the way they were designed. These muscles work best with low resistance. If too much resistance is used, the larger mobilizing muscles will try to "out-muscle" the smaller stabilizers, bypassing the training of these incredibly important, often forgotten muscles.[6,7,8]

When talking about the low back, most people think about the muscles that you can see on either side of your spine. Place your hand on either side of your lumbar spine. On each side of it, you will first feel a little valley and then a large muscle, which is actually a collection of muscles called your erector spinae, the mobilizers of the spine. These are the muscles that feel so good when you receive a massage. They are often quite tight and can limit your range of motion.

However, these are *not* the muscles we want to talk about right now.

Move your fingertips into that valley between the spine and the erectors (see figure 1.3*a*). You've now located the spinal stabilizers. Stand up and find that valley just off your spine again (see figure 1.3*b*). Lean forward slightly until you feel this space bulge up against your fingers (see figure 1.3*c*). That feeling is your spinal stabilizers firing. Did both sides fire at the same time? If they didn't that indicates that you may have some dysfunction in your spinal stabilizers. This forward-leaning motion will be reintroduced in the exercise section and I will explain how to get them firing together again.

Your spinal stabilizers are the most important muscles of the spine. These muscles are nearest to the spine; in fact, they lie right on it and hold it together through activity and movement. These muscles have multiple responsibilities, which is to both allow *and* restrict movement. They govern the amount of movement your spine is allowed, and at the same time, can assist the larger muscles in performing a particular range of motion.

The spine has a limited range of motion based on its given structure and biomechanics. The disc, for instance, can only move so far without causing

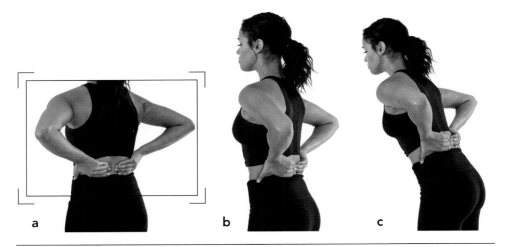

FIGURE 1.3   Finding and assessing your spinal stabilizers.

damage to itself. The bones, likewise, are restricted because too wide a range of motion can lead to damage and injury. The spinal stabilizers are responsible for limiting these motions. They are also responsible for returning the bones back to their original position. Like a spring on a door that slams shut after it's been opened, these muscles restore the spine to its proper position.

The spinal stabilizers are made up of four different muscles: interspinalis, intertransversarii, rotatores, and multifidus (see figure 1.4). They work together to create an interconnected web-like structure, connecting one vertebra to another while allowing some movement.

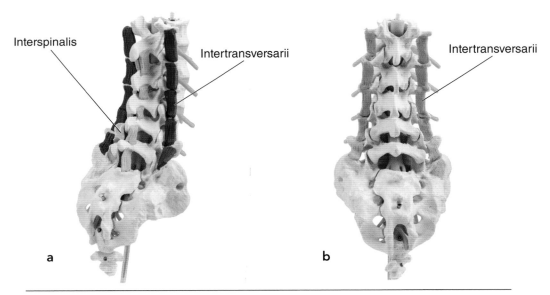

FIGURE 1.4   Spinal stabilizers: *(a)* interspinalis, *(b)* intertransversarii.
Images © Balanced Body Inc. Used with kind permission.

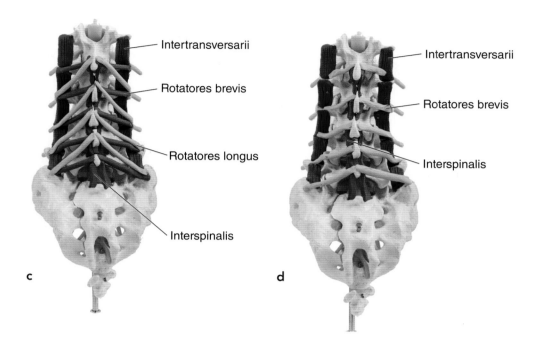

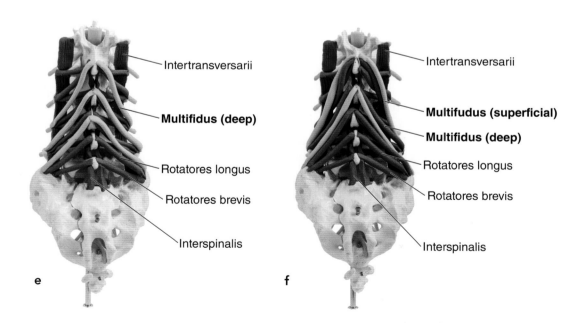

FIGURE 1.4   Spinal stabilizers: *(c)* rotatores longus, *(d)* rotatores brevis, *(e)* deep multifidus, and *(f)* superficial multifidus.

Images © Balanced Body Inc. Used with kind permission.

Interspinalis

The deepest layer of the spinal stabilizers is the interspinalis (see figure 1.4a). This muscle connects from the superior (top vertebra) spinous process to the adjacent spinous process below and is seen primarily in the cervical and lumbar regions of the spine. When the interspinalis fires, it helps to extend and stabilize the spine.

Intertransversarii

The intertransversarii runs in pairs on both sides of your spine from the superior transverse process to the one below, and is found primarily in the cervical and lumbar region (see figure 1.4b). When both sides contract, it stabilizes the spine and assists in extending it. If only one side fires, it assists with side bending (lateral flexion).

Rotatores

The rotatores are made up of two sections called the longus and brevis, meaning long and short (see figure 1.4 c and d). This muscle travels from the spinous process of the superior vertebra (e.g., L1) to the transverse process of the next two vertebrae (L2 and L3). It looks like a wide A. This muscle is most prominent in the thoracic spine, though some literature shows it also in the lumbar spine. Its job is to support the spine and assist in extension and rotation.

Multifidus

The multifidus gets the most attention. People often mention this muscle when they are referring to all the spinal stabilizers. It's easy to see why; the multifidus has the largest surface area of the spinal stabilizers, which means it is easiest to see and easiest for researchers to study. This muscle, like the rotatores, starts at the spinous process of one vertebra (L1) and goes down two, three, and four levels (L3, L4, and L5). This muscle is present from the second cervical vertebra (C2) all the way down the spine. It is a primary stabilizer but also assists in spinal extension, lateral flexion, and rotation.

All of the spinal stabilizer muscles, and the multifidus specifically, support your posture and have a large number of slow-twitch muscle fibers. However, the multifidus has the added distinction of consisting of quite a large amount of fast-twitch fibers.[5] Figure 1.4e shows the deep multifidi spanning two levels which are assumed to have more slow-twitch muscle fibers and less fast-twitch muscle fibers. Figure 1.4f spans three levels which is a more superficial portion and presumed to have more fast twitch muscle fibers. The slower twitch muscles help you to maintain posture for long periods of time and allow you to maintain and return to correct spinal position throughout everyday activities. Without them, the spine would be quite fragile and at greater risk of injury. The fast-twitch fibers are automatic fibers that are responsible for being able to set and reset the spine quickly without any thought. Think of it as a safety mechanism to keep your spine aligned, similar to the steering wheel of a car; when you have made a turn and let the steering wheel go, it will basically return to its starting position. Now imagine that occurring within the blink of an eye. The signal goes from the brain to the muscles almost instantaneously. This occurs so that when you are doing some movement, no matter the speed, your spine stays properly supported and aligned. Problems arise when there is dysfunction in this mechanism and it isn't firing or it is firing too slowly.

A relevant example of dysfunction in this mechanism can be provided by my father. He was walking through a parking garage and inadvertently hit his shoulder against the mirror of an SUV. It turned his body abruptly, and his back spasmed. If his spine had been completely healthy it would have rotated and returned with no ill effects. However, these fast-twitch muscles occasionally forget their job. Their timing slows down and more resembles a slow-twitch muscle. Instead of firing immediately to protect his spine from the sudden rotation, it fired late and his spine was out of position when it contracted, which led to the spasm. He had some existing spinal issues that had gone undiagnosed for years, but this was the proverbial straw that broke the camel's back (no pun intended).

With age and injury, the fast-twitch musculature of the multifidus tends to slow. In fact, when we have an injury to a specific portion of the spine, that specific area can become dysfunctional. These spinal stabilizers are segmentally innervated, meaning that the nerves that innervate them come out of the spinal canal directly at the muscles. So the muscles that support and protect the area of L3 to L4, for example, can become dysfunctional while the rest of the spine may be just fine. We often call the body a kinetic chain, all the segments linking to and communicating with the others. This dysfunctional area becomes the weak link in our chain, and once dysfunctional, it can be a challenge to reactivate the area, to wake it up so to speak and remind the muscles of their job.

Why are these muscles so important? Well, imagine a tent. The tent is held up by tent poles that are attached to ropes staked into the ground. If all the ropes are taut and pulling equally on the tent poles, the tent will be able to withstand the forces of wind and rain. These ropes make the tent stable. If we cut one or two of the ropes, the tent will probably still stand, but the structural integrity will be substantially weakened; a big gust of wind will collapse it. Your body functions like the tent: The tent poles are the spine that provide the structural support, and the ropes are the spinal stabilizers that hold the tent poles in place and give them increased strength and support. So, the muscles to focus on when working with spinal and core stability are these spinal stabilizers.

Mobilizers of the Spine

If the deep muscles are responsible for stabilizing the spine, it is the more superficial muscles that are the mobilizers. These muscles allow you to move freely and achieve your spine's maximum range of motion. After working in the fitness industry for over 25 years, I am amazed at how many people still think that the larger and stronger the muscle, the less flexible it is. Most people picture the big bodybuilder type of guy and assume he has a hard time moving around because he is so "muscle-bound." The opposite is usually true. Some of the most flexible people I know are athletes who have a lot of muscle.

Unfortunately, however, these muscles also have a tendency toward dysfunction, which usually means weakening and tightening. The mobilizing muscles that affect the low back and contribute to pain and injury are the hip flexors, hamstrings, erectors, quadratus lumborum, and gluteus maximus (see figure 1.5).

Hip Flexors

Your hip flexors are comprised of two muscles that originate in different areas and merge at a common insertion point on the thigh (see figure 1.5a). The first muscle is the psoas. It originates on your lumbar spine, attaching to the transverse processes and bodies of the vertebrae, then running diagonally through the pelvis. The iliacus, the second muscle, originates on the front side of your ilium (hip bone) and meets up with the psoas after they exit the pelvis and attach to the femur (thigh bone). These muscles are responsible for flexing your hip as well as tipping your hip forward into an anterior tilt. This dynamic duo of hip flexion is notorious for becoming tight. When it becomes tight, it often tilts your pelvis forward, resulting in an increased lordosis, or lumbar curve, putting increased compression on to the lumbar vertebrae and the discs.

Hamstrings

Most people are familiar with the hamstrings. They are located on the backs of the thighs and connect the lower leg (below the knee) with the hip (see figure 1.5b). The hamstrings are a group of muscles that span two joints, both the knee and hip. They are not only responsible for bending the knee but also for extending the hip. This is very important for us in gait (walking). With each step, the hamstrings (and glutes) contract to bring the leg back behind the body to propel you forward. These muscles can also become tight and weak. When they tighten up, we see that they contribute to tipping the pelvis forward, an anterior pelvic tilt, which, again, increases lordosis and pressure on the discs.

Erector Spinae

The erector spinae are the group of muscles that come to mind when you think of the low back and low back pain. They are the big muscles on either side of your spine (see figure 1.5c). They are comprised of three sets of muscles that allow you to arch and side-bend your spine. Unfortunately, these muscles tend to tighten up after an injury, which leads to an exaggerated lumbar

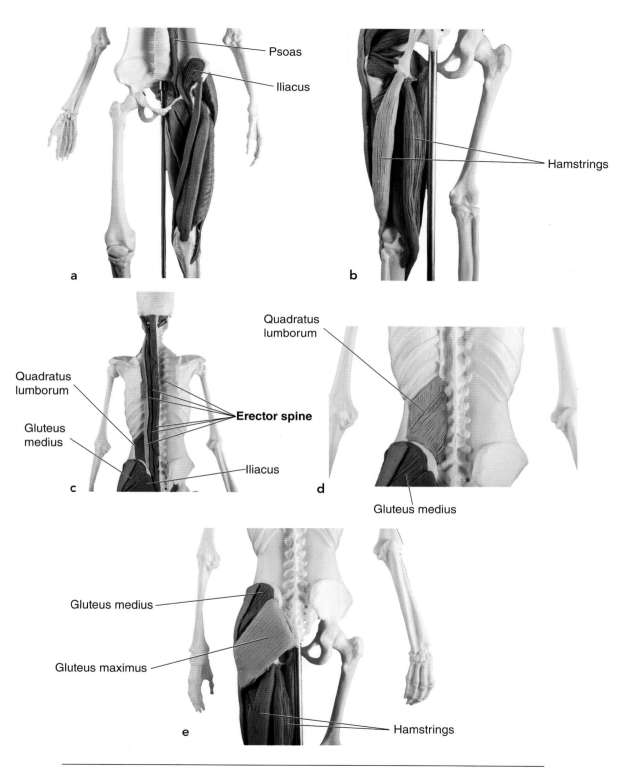

FIGURE 1.5   Spinal mobilizers: *(a)* hip flexors, *(b)* hamstrings, *(c)* erector spinae, *(d)* quadratus lumborum, and *(e)* gluteus maximus.
Images © Balanced Body Inc. Used with kind permission.

curve (lordosis) that increases compression of the discs. These are muscles that need to be supple and flexible, yet after a low back injury, they can seize up and become very stiff and inflexible.

Quadratus Lumborum

This muscle is the workhorse of the lumbar spine. The quadratus lumborum (QL) is a wide and multilayered muscle that runs from the lowest rib to the hip bone (ilium) with branches attaching to the transverse processes of the lumbar vertebrae (see figure 1.5d). This muscle allows for side bending as well as extension (back bending). It is active any time your low back is in motion. Anytime you sit, stand, or walk, it contracts to move your spine. It also happens to be a muscle that can cause pain. When it gets too stiff, it can pull on your pelvis and cause problems with your sacroiliac joint, which is where the bottom of your spine, the sacrum, attaches to the pelvis (ilium). Often referred to as your SI joint, it can be a contributing factor to lower back pain. This pain is often due to instability of the SI joint, and can manifest itself as numbness, tingling, or radiating pain down the leg. This may be one of the factors when someone is diagnosed with sciatica.

Straight Talk

Sciatic nerve pain, often called sciatica, is usually referred to as numbness, tingling, or radiating pain down the leg. But sciatica is more of a symptom rather than a diagnosis. There are multiple conditions that can cause sciatic nerve pain: a disc issue (herniation or bulge), SI joint dysfunction, spondylolisthesis, subluxation, piriformis syndrome, or stenosis. It is vitally important that you understand the actual medical diagnosis to properly manage your condition. Please don't guess. Spinal exercises are specific to your condition, and certain exercises may be contraindicated for you. Ask your physician or physical therapist to diagnose your condition before doing the exercises given later in this book.

Gluteus Maximus

Next we focus on your gluteus maximus: your rear, butt, tush, badonkadonk (see figure 1.5e). Whatever you want to call it, your glutes need to be a lot stronger than they currently are. As we age, we tend to see atrophy of our gluteal muscles. They lose strength and size. Think about an elderly man: how many do you know with large, well-defined glutes? Unless they are a high-level athlete, I can't think of any. We need to preserve these muscles at all costs.

There is another reason we need to train them. With lower back pain, we often see these muscles shut down to a significant degree. I'm not sure who coined these phrases but I've seen the phenomenon called dormant butt syndrome or gluteal amnesia. The glutes either shut off or delay firing. This pattern can lead to the erectors becoming hypertonic, or overactive, meaning they fire all the time even when they aren't supposed to. That back spasm you've felt? It could be a by-product of your erectors or QLs being overactive or hyperactive. In that situation, the glutes shut down.

I recall a client doing a glute-specific exercise, and I could see that her glutes weren't firing. I had her place her hands on her rear end and tell me if she felt the muscles contracting. She was floored; they weren't contracting at all. It actually took a few weeks to turn those muscles back on. Personally, when I've injured my back in the past, trying to wake up these muscles has been a real chore. It often takes a few exercise sessions before they wake up and begin to fire again.

The Spinal Unit

Most people think of the spine as a singular object. We call it our spine or spinal column, don't we? But the spine is actually comprised of 25 individual joints (not including the coccyx) from top to bottom, and that only accounts for the vertebra to vertebra connections. In the thoracic region, you also have joints where the ribs attach, but that is for another book and another day. Each of these joints is made up of the top and bottom vertebra and the disc that sits between them. This is referred to as the spinal unit.

Understanding the spinal unit is important, especially when we begin talking about low back pain and specific spinal conditions. In looking at the spinal unit, you can see that each vertebra creates a joint that, depending on its spinal region, can rotate, and flex forward, back, and side to side. It also absorbs compressive (pushing together), tension (pulling apart), and shear (sliding) forces. Placing these spinal units together produces a spine that is strong and resilient yet still susceptible to injury.

We should mention something about "neutral spine" and spinal "bias." I have had the pleasure of teaching thousands of fitness professionals for over 15 years. A question I ask that seems to stump the students is, "What is neutral spine?" The reason it stumps people is that, depending on the area of the fitness industry they are in, neutral spine may have different definitions. Pilates, yoga, bodybuilding, and general fitness professionals may all have slightly different ways to describe this concept.

The traditional definition that I learned years ago is that neutral spine is the posture of your pelvis in which the anterior superior iliac spine is in line with the posterior superior iliac spine. I probably just lost you, as most people have no idea what that means. Someone who has studied anatomy may understand this definition but it may not mean anything to the average person.

To help understand neutral spine, let's demonstrate it. Lie down on the floor. Note how your low back feels on the ground. Do you have a high arch to your back, the sort of arch where a chihuahua could walk under it? Okay, to get to a more neutral state, flatten out your lumbar spine a bit. Think of the arch in your lumbar as a small foot bridge rather than the Golden Gate

Bridge. On the other extreme, if your back is pressed completely flat to the ground, that is too flat. You need to have a slight arch in your spine. So, the rule of thumb upon lying down is that you want a small arch to your back as long as it doesn't cause you discomfort or pain. That is your neutral spine. If it does cause you some pain, then find the position you can maintain without discomfort. For your body, that becomes your neutral spine. Even though it may not be the true definition of neutral spine, for your body, it is neutral. Over time, you may find that you are able to get closer to the traditional definition. This is called your bias.

Your directional preference, or pelvic bias, is the position of your pelvis relative to your lumbar spine that causes no additional pain or relieves pain symptoms. Some people feel better in a flat-back position; we call this spinal flexion or posterior pelvic tilt (see figure 1.6a). Other people prefer to be in more of an extended position with a larger arch to their spine; we call this spinal extension or anterior pelvic tilt (see figure 1.6b). Whichever position feels better for your body is your preference or bias. In fact, depending on your specific medical condition, you may need to exercise in your preferred bias in order to avoid pain. This preferred bias is your neutral spine.

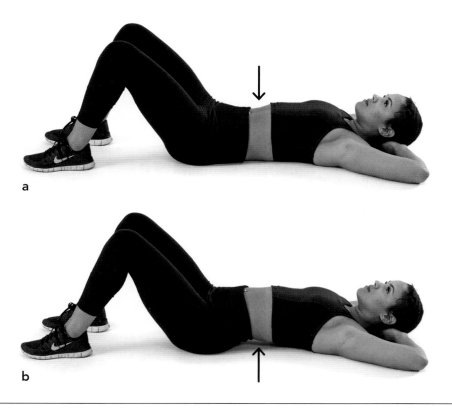

FIGURE 1.6 Pelvic bias: (a) spinal flexion (flat back) or (b) spinal extension (low back arch).

It's important to be able to find your neutral spine because it is the safest and typically the most comfortable position for your spine. This is the position in which your spine should bear the least amount of stress and strain, and experience the least amount of pull from the effects of gravity and muscular tension. Unfortunately, most of us have developed bad postural habits over time that have altered our spine, and our posture begins to resemble a question mark.

Gravity pulls the upper body forward into a rounded posture. Muscular imbalances and tight muscles can exacerbate this, and soon this poor posture becomes permanent. It isn't confined to a single spinal region; it can and often does affect your entire spine.

When you lose your neutral spine in one area (e.g., lumbar), its effects are carried all along the spine. Like a chain reaction, when one region deviates from its neutral position, it results in an altered posture for the rest of the spine. Have you ever heard the phrase, "Where the head goes, the body follows"? It's true when it comes to posture. As your head drops forward (protracts), your thoracic spine (midback) begins to round forward, as do your shoulders. This leads to your lumbar spine increasing its curve, or its lordosis, as well, which increases compressive forces on the discs. Maintaining your neutral spine during exercise will help take stress off your discs and begin to slowly improve your posture. See figure 1.7 for an example of proper and poor posture.

One way for you to begin to reverse the effects of gravity and poor daily posture is to work on finding and maintaining a neutral spine throughout the day. Try this while at work. Set an alarm for every hour. When it goes off, adjust your posture and try to maintain it for 60 seconds. While it may seem that isn't enough time to really accomplish anything, remember this is just a starting point. For some people, holding good posture is so foreign that it will be very difficult to maintain for even a minute. You can slowly begin to adjust the times on both your alarm and the duration of hold. Hold the posture for 75 seconds then 90 seconds and so on. Then begin to adjust the alarm to every 50 minutes instead of every hour. You can reduce this to every 10 minutes if you choose. The important thing to remember is that this exercise has two goals. The first is to make you conscious of your posture. Most of us are so unconscious of it that we don't ever give it a thought, so just making yourself aware of it is a great place to start. The second goal is the importance of reminding and training these muscles to recall the optimal position. With practice, your muscles will begin to get stronger and have more endurance to hold you in the proper position for longer periods of time.

So now that you know everything there is to know about the anatomy of the spine, you are ready to dive headlong into the exercises, right? Not so fast. Remember that this is an introduction to spinal anatomy. You have the basics to move on to the next section in which we begin to discuss the importance of spinal stabilization. We will focus on what that is and how to regain the natural stabilizing forces your spine had once upon a time, before it was injured. It's these spinal stabilization techniques and exercises that will help you to rebuild your spine and create the support it needs for daily life.

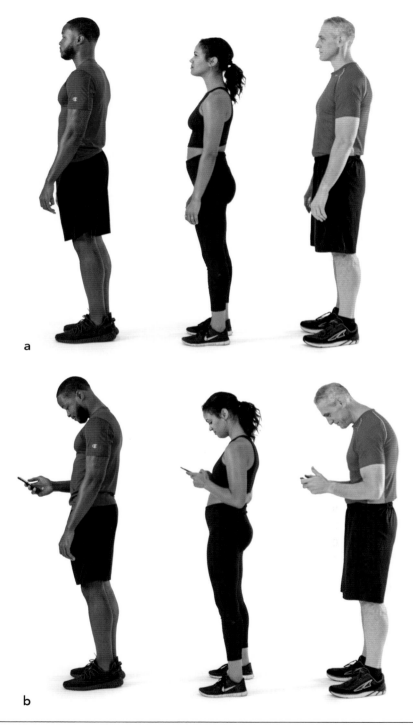

FIGURE 1.7   Shown here are (a) a variety of average postures and (b) a variety of poor postures.

CHAPTER 2

Spinal Stability Training

Now that you know why it's so important to train these spinal muscles and keep them strong, how do you do it? Most exercise focuses on what is moving, but this training is, at least in the beginning, all about what *isn't* moving. Later in the book, I teach you some exercises and your instinct is going to be to focus on the moving parts. I'm going to ask you to do the opposite.

I want you to focus that attention on your spine and core and keeping them still. You should not roll your hips, or arch and flatten your back. It is vitally important that throughout these exercises you keep your spine and core motionless. That being said, I do not want you to "brace" using your muscles, which is a technique often taught at the beginning of the rehab process as a way to keep your core tight and your spine stable. It is very appropriate to use this technique during the beginning stages of rehab when your body doesn't know what to do, and your spine is unstable and moving in ways that are inefficient or worse yet, problematic. You need to retrain the spinal stabilizers to remember their job and to become efficient at it. However, if you continue to brace all the time, it will ultimately lead to inefficient movement patterns and the development of bad habits. I want to train your body for daily life. Imagine trying to walk while holding your abdominals as tightly as you can, and maintaining this. Can you walk normally? I can't. And that's just walking. Imagine trying to do activities of daily life in that position. It simply can't be done, at least not for extended periods of time. Talk about tiring out those muscles!

Instead, you want to train these muscles to fire when they need to, automatically, and to let go when not needed. This will make them much more efficient in doing their job properly. After an injury, people often excessively brace the muscles as a way to avoid pain. This strategy may have some benefit at the very beginning, during the acute stage of injury, but doing this too much may create a bad habit that can linger for years or even decades. I want to make sure you're not instilling that habit. You need to stay stable, but not be clenching your muscles for dear life. Golfers have a great analogy when talking about gripping their golf club. Imagine you are holding a baby bird.

Hold it firm enough so that it doesn't fly away but not so tight that you hurt it. The same applies to your spinal stabilizers.

Remember that all of your muscles have a specific job for which they were designed. Unfortunately, when we are injured, many other muscles try to assist, whether they are designed to do so or not. We need to remind these muscles of their primary job and have them focus on that. Think of your muscles as a new employee: anxious to help out where they can and to do whatever is necessary to help. It seems like a nice idea, but that person can soon get in the way. I want to train your muscles to be more like a union laborer. They have one job that they do well and they have no interest in doing anyone else's job for them.

Building Spinal Stability

My first introduction to spinal stabilization exercise came over 20 years ago from physical therapist Michael Jones, PhD, of the American Academy of Health Fitness and Rehab Professionals. Dr. Jones teaches spinal stability in three stages: fully supported, partially supported, and then unsupported. We

Commonly Asked Questions About Spinal Stabilization

I was first introduced to the concept of the "core" being more than just abdominal muscles from one of my university professors, Dr. Jan Prins. He asked us, "How many of you train your abs?" All hands went up. Then he asked, "How many of you train your lower back muscles?" About half the class kept their hands up. Then he asked us, "How many of you train the lumbar muscles with the same number of sets and reps as your abs?" No hands were left raised. This was in the '90s before the concept of core training. It was called ab training and it usually consisted of doing crunches.

So much has changed in the past several decades in how we view and train our core. For many people, it still involves a lot of crunches and maybe some planks, but this limits the focus to the abs. I want you to think about going much deeper to the spinal stabilizers because it is those muscles that need to get stronger in order to support your spine. You may have some questions about spinal stability and I hope that I address them in this chapter. To start, here are the most common questions I get about spinal and core stability training.

Why should I focus on stabilizing my spine?
The simple answer is that unless your spine is stable, you won't be able to move well. Remember that your spine is actually a combination of 25 joints. Each has to be stable and doing its job properly in order to have efficient and effortless movement. If the spine isn't stable, there will be improper movement that will cause issues.

How long will it take?
My answer is always the same, "It depends." Every body is different and every condition is different. Sometimes we don't know the answer until we are much further down the road, and each step can change the end point. Another consideration is,

will follow a similar sequence, but will add an all-important fourth stage called dynamic stability, creating a progression from rehabilitation to real life. This systematic progression takes you from a place of your body feeling safe and supported by the structure you're exercising on, all the way up to performing activities of daily life unassisted. That is our goal, first and foremost, to get you back to where you can perform your daily activities with little-to-no discomfort. We will be going over specific exercises and where they fit into the spinal stability spectrum in chapters four through seven. In the chapters that follow, we will break down which exercises are best for specific spinal conditions and diagnoses, and create a six-month workout plan for you to follow to progress from fully supported all the way up to dynamic.

Fully Supported

The first stage of training is fully supported (see figure 2.1). This means that your entire body, or the majority of it, is supported by the ground, a table, or maybe even a bed (although a bed is not the best choice because the softness may inhibit some of the exercises). The goal is to have a lot of surface contact

"How consistent are you working to get better?" I hear it all the time, "I am doing my exercises just like you asked me to." But when I dig deep, it is similar to when the dentist asks you about the last time you flossed your teeth. Some people aren't doing enough to see progress as quickly as they would like.

How often do I need to do the exercises?
Consistency is key to making progress. I recommend doing the exercises every day. Yes, I do realize that may seem unrealistic, but hear me out. When I say do them every day, I know that there will be a day or two that you simply won't have time. Things come up, I get it. But if you strive for every day, I know you will probably get to it three to four times a week. As Norman Vincent Peale said, "Shoot for the moon. Even if you miss, you'll land among the stars." Work hard to do the exercises at least three to four days a week and you'll be more likely to see quicker progress. If you do them all seven days, even better.

When can I stop doing these exercises?
As soon as you want the pain to return. Yes, I am being a little bit of a smart aleck, but in truth, it does come down to that. I was talking with a friend who had just returned to the gym after being out with a shoulder injury for six months. We talked about his rehab and the exercises he had to do every day. He offered this to me: "If by doing these exercises, I never have pain in my shoulder like that again, I will keep doing them." The same goes for the exercises I am going to teach you. They need to be done consistently and for the rest of your life, most likely. I'm sure that sounds overwhelming, but consider the alternative. If you can keep pain at bay by doing 15 to 30 minutes of exercise three times a week, isn't it worth it?

while lying down so that your body doesn't have to stabilize itself for balance or additional support. This support makes it much easier to perform the exercises because your focus can be on maintaining stability and not working to stabilize or balance your body in space.

Most people feel the safest and most comfortable in this stage. Their body feels supported and they feel more confident doing the exercises. You also want to ensure that you are relatively pain-free during these exercises. These are going to be your basic exercises, but they won't be necessarily easy. In this stage, it is very important to focus on keeping your spine still. Do not let your back arch, flatten, or twist during the exercises. Focus on what isn't moving, not what is. We will delve into the specific exercises of fully supported spinal stability in chapter 4.

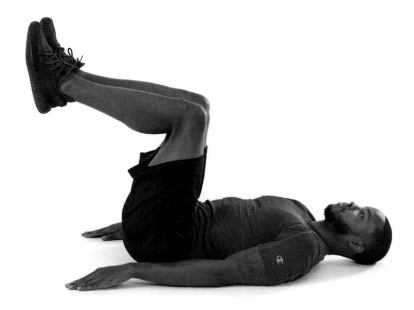

FIGURE 2.1 Tabletop is an example of a fully-supported position.

The second stage of training is partially supported (see figure 2.2). You could be on your hands and knees or seated in a chair with back support. In this way, your body still has a lot of contact with the ground or chair but some additional stability is required while maintaining proper form and posture.

Any time you reduce contact with the ground or supporting surface, the exercise becomes more challenging. We often refer to this as the number of points of contact. If you are on all fours (hands and knees), you have four small points of contact with the ground, unlike when you are lying on your back, in which you have one very large amount of surface contact (the entirety of your backside). Think of a car driving on four tires. There is only a small portion of the tires that is in contact with the ground, yet the car is stable around turns because it is balanced on all four corners.

What happens when you remove one of the points of contact? From the all-fours position, if you lift one hand off the ground, you are more unstable and your body requires additional muscular support in order to maintain its original position. The muscles of your spine are asked to engage to a greater degree in order to accomplish the task. In chapter 5 you will find the exercises that fall into the category of partially supported.

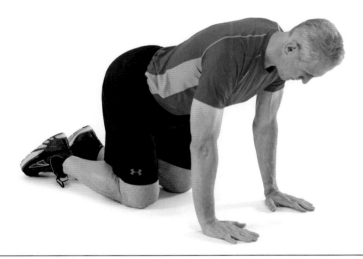

FIGURE 2.2   Quadruped is an example of a partially-supported position.

Unsupported

The third stage of training is unsupported (see figure 2.3). This can be done on a stool with no back support, on a stability ball, or standing—anything that increases the level of stability required by your body while performing the exercise. At this level, there are even fewer points of contact with the ground or surface. In addition, because you are in an upright position, you have to align yourself with gravity and ground forces, which advances you toward activities of daily life. Very few people spend the entire day lying down or on their hands and knees, so you eventually need to get off the ground and learn how to stabilize in the upright position. You also need the ability to stand with your feet in a variety of positions, all while maintaining a neutral spine. For example, have you ever pulled open a freezer door in the supermarket and it feels like the magnetic seal weighs a ton? Obviously, a vacuum was created from within the freezer, but the effect on your body forces you to stabilize from your feet all the way to your hand in order to open that freezer door.

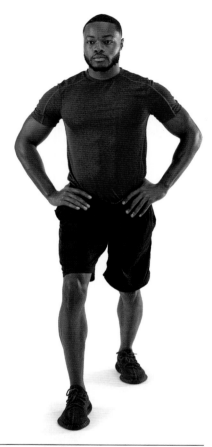

FIGURE 2.3 Standing is an example of an unsupported position.

The ability to plant yourself and stabilize the body is this third level. In chapter 5 we demonstrate the exercises for unsupported spinal stability.

This is where ground forces come into play as well. You are planting yourself into the ground in order to stabilize your core and body to perform a particular action. In sports, one of the best examples of this is a baseball pitcher. If you look at today's pitchers, they all have well-developed legs and glutes, much more developed than their upper body. The reason for this is that they're generating a great amount of force and power with each pitch, starting at the ground and moving up through the entire body. Nearly all power comes from their legs; their arms are just the end of the motion, used more for ball spin and trajectory. The power comes from the force their body exerts against the ground. Now apply that analogy to opening the freezer at the supermarket. If you don't plant your legs first, you won't be able to generate any power.

Dynamic

The final stage of training is dynamic. This is the body in full motion. The ability to stabilize your spine while in motion applies to all the exercise you do in everyday life. I have clients who can't walk up a flight of stairs without their backs hurting. They need to learn how to stabilize their spine and maintain this stability while going from floor to floor, or when walking down the street or getting up off the floor. All these movements are dynamic; you are moving your body through space and need to be stable in order to do this with less discomfort or pain.

Straight Talk

I am often asked to distinguish the differences between performing exercises from seated, standing, or lying down. Think about what is supporting you to maintain your body's posture. While lying down, you need the least amount of additional support to maintain the correct position. While seated, you need the muscles of your hips, spine, core, scapula or shoulders, and neck. A standing position requires you to stabilize your glutes, quadriceps, hamstrings, calves, and feet. The further away from the supporting surface, the more muscles that are required to maintain proper form. Finally, we progress to increasingly more dynamic exercises that require the most spinal stability, and also mimic real life. Without working in each body position and gradually creating sufficient stability and strength in our spinal stabilizers, injury would most likely be the eventual outcome.

Increasing Spinal Stability

Once these muscles are stronger, you need to work on endurance, referred to as tissue tolerance. Muscles can perform a certain number of repetitions for a certain amount of time while maintaining their stability before they fatigue and say, "I'm outta here! Please, someone else, help me do my job." That's when you begin to compensate by using other muscles that weren't designed to do the job now being asked of them. These adjacent muscles can only tolerate so much before they shut down.

When you take a walk, how long or how far can you go before you start to ache? Maybe you feel fine for the first 20 minutes or for the first mile, but after 30 minutes or a mile and a half, your back starts to hurt. Your spinal stabilizers and glutes are fatigued. The glutes should be one of the primary movers in walking, and the spinal stabilizers should keep your spine supported with each step. Your erector spinae and quadratus lumborum are now forced to do the job of the other groups, which becomes a primary cause of low back pain. Again, it is not their job to propel your body to walk. That is why you need to train these muscles to do their designated job and develop a higher tissue tolerance so that the muscles that are not designed to support these activities are not pushed toward injury.

The goal is to increase your strength so you can perform activities for increasingly longer periods of time. You may notice that your back begins to ache around one o'clock in the afternoon every day. The muscles of your back have had enough and they are sending signals that they are done. That is all the endurance they have in them. The goal is for this amount of time to increase. After a few weeks of consistent exercises, you may notice your back doesn't ache until three o'clock, then five o'clock, or on your way home from work. Eventually you want to have enough endurance to last the entire day with no aches or pain. But this process takes time and work. So be patient and diligent.

Let's talk about volume of exercises, repetitions, and sets. Doing only one set of one or two exercises probably won't get the job done. Sorry to break it to you, but you have to put in the work if you want the results. You need to do multiple sets of each exercise in order for your body to respond with an increase in strength and endurance, and hopefully a reduction in discomfort and pain. I have a physical therapist friend who told me she was always searching for the one perfect exercise that would work on everyone. The problem is, it doesn't exist. You need to exercise the muscles from a variety of positions and angles, and perform a lot of sets and reps.

The muscles you are working are referred to as postural muscles, a term which has multiple definitions. Yes, they are partially responsible for keeping you erect and having better posture; however, the definition I am using describes their makeup. Vladimir Janda, often referred to as the father of rehabilitation, divided our muscles into two systems, phasic and postural or tonic. Phasic muscles are built for movement. They are often (though not exclusively) fast-twitch muscles that tend toward weakness when injured. Postural or tonic muscles are generally slower, twitch-oriented, and built for endurance.[1] But no muscle exists in a vacuum acting independently; the two groups often work in a cocontraction to stabilize the joint during movement by balancing the muscles affecting the joint, allowing it to move properly.

Our postural muscles are built to hold our body upright against the force of gravity for long periods of time. These are super-endurance muscles that need to be trained as such. They need a higher number of exercises, sets, and reps; the more the better for these muscles. Begin with three to four exercises and perform two to three sets to start. As you become more proficient in performing these exercises, add new ones until you are performing between 15 to 25 sets of exercises per session. I am a firm believer in higher repetitions. Begin with 10 and work up to 30 reps per exercise. Remember that these are endurance muscles; they respond best to low intensity and high volume. There are also some exercises that will involve an isometric hold for 5 to 10 seconds, creating a sustained muscular contraction to effect a long-lasting change.

The exercises for our postural or stabilizing muscles should be performed at a relatively slow pace. You will know you are performing them correctly when you have a feeling of "chattering," a vibrating or shaking in the limb or muscle. This often indicates that these stabilizing muscles are weak or unaccustomed to the specific exercise. Most people have a tendency to speed up the exercises, which can bypass the smaller stabilizer muscles and cause the larger muscle groups to take over and overpower the smaller muscles. The smaller muscles are meant to do the majority of the work, so perform them slow and controlled. When you get that chattering in the muscle, you'll know you are on the right track.

It is important to note that you may feel some discomfort while doing the spinal stabilizing exercises. Most people don't, but you may, which is both okay and not okay. You need to respect where your body is today. A general rule of thumb is to stay within a pain-free range of motion throughout all your exercises. However, if you have slight discomfort, perhaps a 2 or a 3 on the pain scale (where 1 is no pain and 10 is the worst possible pain), that's okay to work through for two to four repetitions, but don't do more than that. If you are able to do only a few repetitions of each exercise to start, that's fine. It's simply a starting point. Next week, you'll likely be able to do a few more, and then a few more after that. That's how you get stronger and build your muscular endurance. Above all else, listen to your body. If it is signaling you to stop, please do. There is no reason to push through to the point of pain. One of my mentors, Dr. Michael Jones, often reminded us that "No one ever died of acute lack of exercise." When in doubt, leave it out. This goes for all exercises.

Understanding Spinal Stability Training Types

I have explained spinal stability training, so now I want to talk a bit about the other training methods that you should be doing as well. These are especially important once you begin to feel better, have greater function, and feel you can do more with your body without pain.

Core Work

Many people think that spinal stability training is just core work. In reality, the two are very different, yet very important. They each have their role to play in managing low back pain. Spinal stability work involves what isn't moving. Your focus is on keeping your spine still while other parts of your body are in motion. Core work often involves movement of the trunk, but it may also be engaged in some of the spinal stability exercises discussed later, such as planks. Classic exercises that fit into this category would be crunches and bicycles.

It's important to include these core exercises during the dynamic level of spinal stability training as well as afterward, when you begin to mainstream your training into a more general fitness routine. These core exercises act as a bridge to functional activities and activities of daily life. It is foolish to think that you would need to keep your spine completely still for the rest of your life. Can you imagine trying to remain rigid with absolutely no spine movement? Talk about robotic. No, the goal is to strengthen these stabilizers with specific stabilization exercises, then add in more traditional core work. This is to create a strong core capable of full ranges of motion while supporting the spine throughout your everyday activities.

Think about what you do in the course of a day: all the times you get in and out of the car, sit down and get back up, or bend over to pick something up. On a daily basis we stoop, reach, bend, twist, slouch, and extend multiple times. The spine is meant to handle these motions. It is your job to rebuild these muscles so that you can do the movements without hesitation and worry. After a back injury I often see people walk around "braced," and I'm not talking about wearing a corset. I'm talking about holding everything together so tightly that it restricts normal movement. That will keep your spine safe at the beginning, but you can't expect to do it forever. I want you to be able to move freely, or at least more freely than you might currently be capable of. Core work will be introduced and added into your sessions around month five to six to begin your transition to proper movement patterns. You will eventually move better and under more control with a newfound ability to stabilize your spine, thus keeping you safe while moving more freely.

The only caveat with movement is that based on your currently diagnosed medical condition, you may need to restrict range of motion in certain directions to keep yourself safe (we discuss these conditions later in the book). Many people are able to perform greater ranges of motion with little to no pain as they grow stronger, even with other medical conditions. However, I would still recommend staying as safe as possible when exercising.

Lower-Extremity Training

A strong correlation exists between having a strong spine and strong lower body. Your legs need to get stronger as your spine does. Unfortunately, lower-body training seems to be an area where many people, especially men, fall short. How many times have you seen guys with big muscles in their upper body and relatively small muscles in their lower body? I see it all the time. Why? Leg work isn't as glamorous or as much fun to do as other exercises. Also, it often involves hard work with results that are hidden by a pair of pants instead of shown off through a tight T-shirt.

There are a lot of exercises to consider for working your legs, and I want to give you the biggest bang for your buck. In addition to specific gluteal exercises, these exercises for your lower extremities will often be compound exercises, ones that involve using your legs in a functional manner, and using all your leg muscles at once. Think about a squat compared to a leg extension. The leg extension exercise primarily works the quadriceps muscle (front of the thigh) while the squat works your quadriceps, hamstrings, glute, inner thighs, calves, and even your feet—not to mention all the muscles above the belt line that help to stabilize your trunk. This is an exercise that can be done with or without weights. You do not need to have a huge bar with a lot of weight on your shoulders. Try this: Simply stand up and sit back down again. There you go—that is a squat, and you worked all of those muscles I just mentioned.

There is one lower-body exercise that I am going to caution you from doing in the gym. That exercise is the 45 degree leg press. This is an older machine that has been around for a long, long time. You load weight onto the machine, sit close to the ground, and place your legs up in the air at a 45-degree angle with your feet on a plate. You lower the weight toward you and thrust the weight back up in the air. This machine is the culprit of many a herniated or ruptured disc. Most people use too much weight and, at the bottom of the exercise, they round their back to help get the weight back up. I would avoid this machine. There are some safe leg-press machines out there, but you should consider using your own body as the machine instead. Bodyweight exercises such as the squat, step-up, and lunge are often the best for your body and far more functional for daily life. I will include some of the most valuable exercises for your lower body in the exercise section of the book. Keep in mind though, these are only a sample of exercises you can perform. There are tens of thousands of exercises you can choose from. Just because I don't list them doesn't mean you can't do another exercise that you know and like. By all means add some of your own to my list.

Cardiovascular Conditioning

One of the questions I ask potential clients is, "Has a doctor ever told you not to exercise?" Nearly everyone laughs and says, "Quite the contrary." Or "I wish." I ask this to find out if the client has a contraindication to exercise.

But let's face it, we all need exercise, especially cardiovascular exercise, or aerobic exercise. The main reason is for heart health. Regular cardiovascular activity increases your lung capacity, improves your circulatory system, and keeps your heart (a muscle in its own right) strong and healthy. In fact, the American Heart Association recommends 150 minutes per week, or 30 minutes five times per week.[2]

Another reason to increase your cardiovascular fitness has to do with cellular biology. Your skeletal muscles respond to exercise by increasing both the number and size of the mitochondria.[3] The mitochondria are the powerhouse of your cells that convert the energy from food into cellular energy. The larger and more prolific the mitochondria are within a cell, the better they are able to create energy, and to do so more efficiently. This increased efficiency facilitates better oxygen utilization and can assist the healing process. Regular cardiovascular activity can reduce muscular stiffness, thus increasing the mobility of your lumbar spine, and increase localized circulation to promote healing. Motion is lotion: The more you move the better lubricated your muscles, connective tissue, and joints will be.

The type of cardiovascular activity you choose will depend on your personal preference, tissue tolerance or pain, and access to equipment. We all have a favorite form of aerobic exercise, or at least a most tolerable form if forced to choose. Whether it is walking outside or using the stationary bike at the gym, you need to find the type with which you are most comfortable and are able to do for a prolonged period of time. For most people I recommend walking if their body can tolerate it. Walking is something that most people will be able to do: The cost is a pair of good shoes and exercise clothes. No gym membership and no expensive equipment; for about $100, you can start.

If walking is not an option, then a stationary bike or elliptical machine may be the best option. I highly recommend trying out many brands of equipment, because each brand is made differently. For people who do not fall into the category of average height, five feet four inches to six feet two inches, certain brands may be uncomfortable or may bother your back. Try out a few different brands before giving up; most likely, there is a piece of equipment that will work for you but you might have to search for it. If you are looking to purchase a piece for your home, price does matter. I suggest looking for used, but good quality, cardio equipment. Most sellers will tell you the piece has almost no use and they're getting rid of it because they need the space. You'll be able to purchase a quality piece of equipment for pennies on the dollar.

I suggest starting out with a realistic goal of exercising either four times per week for 20 minutes at a time, or three times per week for 30 minutes. This is a volume that people typically won't argue about; it is reasonable and pretty easy to accomplish. Over the subsequent few months you can slowly increase the amount of time or frequency of sessions. A good goal to work toward is the American Heart Association's recommended 150 minutes per week.

Flexibility and Mobility Training

In an earlier section we discussed spinal range of motion, and more specifically, each region's varying range of motion. Your lumbar spine has the greatest degrees of motion in flexion and extension (forward and backward bending) and lateral flexion (side bending), but not much rotation.

With low back pain, it is common that when the muscles in this region become increasingly stiff there is a tendency to move less. One reason is that when your back is in spasm, moving the wrong way can cause the spasm to occur so you avoid moving altogether. The unfortunate byproduct is that you move less and less and the area freezes up. The connective tissue in your low back becomes incredibly stiff and the ability to bend over or tie your shoes becomes more difficult.

Straight Talk

The connective tissue in your lower back is like a rubber band. A new rubber band is very flexible and supple; it moves and returns to its original shape with ease. It will continue to do so as long as it isn't subjected to negative stress like extreme temperatures or excessive range of motion. But sometimes a rubber band hasn't been used in years. Maybe it is wrapped around some papers in the closet and has become dried and stiff. What happens when you try to remove it? At best, it comes off cracked and stretched way out of shape, without many remaining elastic properties. Worst case scenario, it breaks as soon as you move it. Your connective tissue is much like this rubber band. It wants to be flexible and stay in motion, but we all have a tendency to remain in static positions for long periods and our backs tighten up over time. Remember, motion is lotion. You need to keep moving in order to lubricate your muscles, joints, and connective tissue.

Along with stability training, you need to focus on increasing flexibility. The low back muscles are closely related to your hip flexors, hamstrings, and hip rotators. All of these muscles tend to shorten and weaken when you experience an injury to your low back.[4] In chapter 6, you will find safe stretching exercises that will increase your flexibility over time. And it does take time. It took years to become as stiff as you are; you need to be patient, because becoming more flexible isn't going to happen overnight.

In addition to keeping your lumbar spine flexible and mobile, you should also foster movement in the thoracic spine. The thoracic (midback) region is the area of your torso in which you rotate. As you move less and tighten up in your lower back, there is a corresponding tightness in the thoracic region as well. That lack of mobility in your thoracic spine often takes shape as a kyphosis, a rounding of the shoulders and midback, which reduces the range of motion of extension (being able to stand up and maintain tall posture) and rotation.

Straight Talk

Have you noticed over the years that you aren't able to turn your head and look out the back of your car like you did when you were younger? Often the restriction isn't limited to your neck but also your thoracic spine. The ability to turn your shoulders can be affected as you age and move less. But I do have a quick and easy solution that will help you while driving: Simply lean forward a little and pull your back away from the seat back, then try turning your shoulders and head. You should be able to increase your range of motion significantly. This doesn't solve all the problems of midback tightness, but you will be able to rotate your body to its fullest potential. As you increase flexibility in this area, you will be able to rotate even more.

But recent treatment methods have shown that performing thoracic strengthening and mobility training at the same time as spinal stability training results in a significant increase in strength of the spinal muscles[5] and improved recovery times.

The thoracic spine and hips are designed for rotation, much more so than the lumbar spine. Then why do so many people want to turn through their lumbar spine? One reason is that, over the years, bodies become inflexible in the thoracic spine and hips so the lumbar area wants to help out. This is another example of the lumbar spine wanting to do someone else's job. Add an exercise or two to your routine to begin to train your thoracic spine to move the way it was designed—specifically to increase extension and rotation—while at the same time working on stabilizing the spine and hip mobilization. Getting your hips to move properly is one of the keys to better spinal stability. We will address this with the exercises shown later in the book.

In the past two chapters you've learned about spinal anatomy and the types of exercises you will be performing. Before we jump into the exercises you need to figure out where exactly you are: What is your starting point? In order to do this, the next chapter will provide a self-assessment. This will give you a baseline to compare with as you get stronger, and it will identify any red flags that would indicate you may not be ready to proceed or that you may want to check with your doctor or physical therapist before continuing.

CHAPTER 3

Assess Yourself

Several years ago I was sitting in a seminar with a well-respected lecturer. He asked us a question, and his own answer made me do a double take. He asked, "Do all clients need an assessment?" I was already nodding my head in the affirmative when he said, "No. No, they do not." I couldn't believe my ears. He then went on to tell the class how assessments are a waste of time because any exercise is appropriate for any client. "My grandmother should be able to do the same exercises as my mixed martial arts fighters," he argued. Truthfully, my first thought was, "That is one kick-butt grandma." My next thought was, "Are you crazy?" Needless to say, I left that seminar immediately.

Without a doubt, all clients who walk through my door get an assessment because it provides an opportunity to learn a great deal about them and determine the point from which they are starting. Without a starting point, how will you be able to track progress and know how far you've progressed? Many people expect to jump into exercise on their first session with me, and some professionals may do that depending on the client's condition and other factors. In my opinion, that amounts to malpractice. Until I know everything I can about you, how do I know how to help you achieve your goal? It's similar to wandering around in a dark room looking for a light switch: If you wander around long enough, you will probably find it. But wouldn't it be much easier to know where you are going right from the start? That's exactly where we are going to start, with the assessment.

Pain

"Pain is inevitable. Suffering is optional." I am reminded of this Hindu spiritual quote as I work with clients who suffer with pain. As we age, our bodies break down and pain becomes a part of our lives in one way or another. It is how we accept and deal with this pain that defines us. Some people want to wallow in it while others choose to move past it. We all wish we didn't have the pain, but learning how to manage it is the first step toward moving beyond it.

Over the years I've worked with a large number of people in pain and I have come to understand that pain is very subjective, and a person's tolerance can be anywhere on the map. I've had clients with such high pain tolerance that they don't need Novocain when they go to the dentist. I've also had clients for whom a hangnail consumes their every waking hour, and they are in nonstop agony. I respect each of these scenarios and clients. We all perceive and experience pain in our own way. Before we can work on strengthening the body we must first talk about pain and establish some common vocabulary. Too many people focus only on their pain, which is limiting because success becomes black and white. We don't live in that sort of world; there are a lot of grays and, hopefully, colors too. When it comes to pain, most people say they are either in pain or not. We need to talk about the grades of pains.

Straight Talk

The wife of my client, John, told me something shocking one day: For the last 10 years, every time she and John would see friends, their first question to him was, "How's your back doing?" His back pain had become part of his identity and how he began to think of himself and project himself to others. He was someone with back pain, and constantly focused on his limitations rather than his possibilities.

Managing pain can seem overwhelming, especially when you are in the middle of it. It can be even more overwhelming when you don't know what to do and have no path toward getting better. I'm sure many of you have tried seeing physicians, chiropractors, physical therapists, acupuncturists, or other natural healers. And through all that, you are still in pain.

When it comes to managing pain, you need one thing more than anything else. Belief. You need to maintain a belief that it will get better. I believe that thoughts can become self-fulfilling prophecies. If you believe that you won't get better, guess what? You'll prove yourself correct. On the other hand, if you believe that you will get better and (this is the important part) do everything in your power to get better, you are much more likely to achieve your goal. The next thing you need is a plan, and you may have been given one from your physical therapist or physician, but ask yourself honestly—Have you followed through with it? If you want to get better you need to be committed to your success.

How many times have you heard that an athlete made a remarkable comeback from an injury or surgery that should have sidelined them for an

In medicine, pain is often described as being on a scale from 1 to 10, 1 being very little pain to 10 being extreme pain. A rating of one means that you barely feel anything. A rating of 10 feels like someone is stabbing you. This establishes a common language that everyone will understand.

I was talking to a physical therapist friend about Jim, a client we share. Jim said he was in level 8 pain. My friend and I commented on this because Jim then went on to casually tell us about his weekend, what he did, who he saw, and so on. But his activities and demeanor weren't consistent with his stated pain level. We agreed that if someone were in pain at level 8, they would be breathing heavy, wouldn't be able to get comfortable, and would be unable to concentrate on anything except the pain. While Jim was in some discomfort, it was not a level 8 of pain.

I ask a couple of questions to most of my prospective clients who experience pain. The first question is "What level of pain do you experience on a daily basis?" If they say 6, for instance, I then ask if they would be happy if that fell to a 1 or a 2. Every one of them says, "Yes." Through proper muscle strengthening, there will almost always be an improvement in the pain level. Secondly, I ask, "Would you rather be in pain and feel weak and nonfunctional, or be in pain yet feel strong and functional?" The answer is always the latter. Increasing functionality in life gives you the freedom to do more. Life won't

extended period of time, or worse yet, ended their career, only to see them come back and play even stronger, as though nothing had happened? Are they simply genetically superior to you? Maybe. But they also possessed the desire to get better and a focused determination in knowing that every repetition is one repetition closer to getting back on the field. You have to want it and understand the time commitment involved in getting stronger and building tissue endurance; you have to trust that every exercise session is one step closer to your goal.

No one can do it for you. You have to put in the time and energy.

There is nothing miraculous in this book that guarantees that you will be 100 percent pain-free at the end of it. Success may require managing the pain with exercises for the rest of your life. But you can do it. If doing 30 minutes of exercise four to fives times per week reduces the pain or keeps pain at bay, isn't it worth it?

For John, it took a period of diligent work, but he was able to manage his low back pain with proper exercise to the point it hardly ever bothered him. I can't tell you how happy I was when he said to me, "You know what I just realized? I haven't had any low back pain for nearly a week." At that moment I knew he had turned a corner in his recovery. His attention was no longer so fixated on pain every moment of every day that he could focus on what he could do, rather than what he couldn't do. He could place his attention on his possibilities rather than on his limits. That's when I know someone has managed their pain.

be as limiting, and pain won't be the deciding factor between participating in something you enjoy or staying home and doing nothing. I've seen many people forgo trips with their family or not participate in a function because they are afraid they may end up in more pain. Typically with increased strength and function comes decreased pain.

But no matter where you fall on the pain spectrum, I want you to be honest with yourself about the severity of your back pain. Do you feel mild discomfort or sheer agony? Is it constant or intermittent? Can you find a comfortable position to sit or sleep in, or is that impossible? These are the questions I want you to answer.

I am often asked, "When will I be completely free of pain?" I always answer the same way, "I have no idea." For one thing, I don't know if you will ever be 100 percent free of pain. If that is your goal, I respect it and want to see it happen. But until you travel down that road, you don't know what you will encounter or how long of a journey that will be.

Medical History

As I previously mentioned, every new client who comes through my facility receives an assessment. I want to gather as much information as possible to gain a clear picture of the person with whom I'm working. This information allows me to begin designing an appropriate exercise program for this client.

I want to know as much as I can about their history. All orthopedic issues are important to me, no matter how far in the past they may have occurred. Believe it or not, someone who injured their ankle or knee years previous could now be having back problems partially due to that old injury.

A great example of how a medical history can inform exercise selection is a client, Allie, who suffered from severe knee pain and was scheduled for a double knee replacement. She had been suffering with her knees for years and had put off the replacement surgery as long as she could. Unfortunately for Allie, she was compensating for the knee pain with her low back. Not long after she had her knees replaced, her low back pain increased substantially. For many years, she had walked and climbed stairs any way she could to avoid knee pain, which put increased pressure on her back and caused her to use her low back muscles instead of her leg muscles. Climbing stairs was the worst; to accomplish it she would hoist up her hips instead of bending her knees. It helped to decrease pressure on her knees but the stress it put on her spine was tremendous, as was the back pain she developed because of these modifications. When we have pain, we often alter our normal movement patterns to try to avoid the discomfort; unfortunately, there may be undesirable repercussions because of it. Allie's experience is a relevant example of this.

It is always helpful to know what led to the current pain. Allie's back pain was caused by her knees. When her knees improved she had to deal with her residual lumbar pain. The good news was that her knees wouldn't continue to make her back hurt. Now she could focus solely on her low back and make sure she had good stair climbing mechanics (i.e., using her knees and not her back). However, if she hadn't dealt with her knees, they would have continued to cause her back pain because she would be straining her back in order to avoid increasing the pain in her knees. By knowing her history of knee and low back pain, I was able to properly program her exercise prescription to help manage her current state and condition.

My father's knee provides another example of how understanding a client's medical history can impact a recovery plan. My father tore his meniscus while setting up a Christmas tree. His busy work schedule delayed the repair surgery until June, and in the interim, he developed a pronounced limp that stayed with him long after the surgery. In fact, calf tightness became a major issue because of his limp. All of these issues are connected: Had he come to me as a client with calf tightness and a limp, but not disclose the gap between his initial injury and the surgery, I may have tried to work with components that were not at the root cause of his pain, further delaying his recovery.

Injuries

While talking to clients about their medical history I want a complete account of any injuries. This includes the backstory of what caused an injury and what has been done since. What we often hear is, "I bent over and suddenly couldn't get up" or something similar, but this is, of course, the straw that broke the camel's back, so to speak. Most low back injuries are caused by an accumulation of incidents over a period of time. However, there are times when an acute trauma leads to the injury, such as a car accident, a fall, or some other significant event. This is important to know.

The history of an injury includes but may not be limited to: the proper medical diagnosis, how was the diagnosis made (e.g., MRI, X-ray, muscle testing), the medical procedures or treatments (e.g., surgeries, injections, therapies) undertaken to this point, whether the injury or pain has improved or changed with those treatments and by how much, and the incident that initiated the injury.

Diagnoses

It may be surprising to learn that many people don't know their medical diagnosis. I often hear, "I have low back pain," or "I have sciatica." Only when I press them about the true diagnosis do I begin to uncover the truth. They aren't trying to hide anything, many people simply don't know, or they don't understand what is wrong with them. Unless you are in the medical field, many of these diagnoses can sound like a foreign language. I had a client tell me she had back pain, and she mentioned stenosis. I asked what was done to diagnose it and she said she'd had an MRI. Great, so I asked to see a copy of the results of the MRI; she didn't have it with her but would get it to me. I asked if the

MRI indicated that anything else was wrong. She said no. This is a woman in her mid- to late sixties who wanted to lose weight and had other postural issues that made me question if stenosis was the only issue, but I waited for the MRI. She began performing exercises to manage her stenosis, but with each week she got progressively worse. After three weeks she finally brought in the MRI. The word *anterolisthesis* was recorded, along with stenosis. To her, it was just another word that she didn't recognize or pay attention to. To me, it was the smoking gun. With this new information, we changed her exercises and she immediately began to feel better and to improve. Within weeks, she was in much less pain and able to play golf again. So, it's very important to know and relay your correct diagnosis in order to prescribe and perform the correct exercises.

You may not have a diagnosis yet and if not, I highly recommend you get one. It will usually involve an MRI or X-ray, and most likely both. This can be very important in ensuring you are doing the correct exercises for your body. Keep in mind that going to see an orthopedic surgeon doesn't mean you must have surgery. Surgery is one option for a number of conditions; a good doctor will respect your choice to try physical therapy or to manage the condition through exercise.

Previous Surgeries

Let's talk briefly about surgery. I have had a lot of clients who don't want to go to orthopedic surgeons because "All they want to do is surgery." That is usually not the case; however, remember that surgery is what surgeons do well and it is the biggest tool in their toolbox. They know that they can help you with surgery. But they also know that depending on the severity of your condition there may be other options to explore first. A good physician will exhaust all other options before doing surgery.

Before you jump into surgery, remember that it often permanently and structurally changes the body. Whether removing bone, fusing vertebrae, or something equally invasive, the surgeon is changing the structure of your spine for life. While that may be the only option, I would try all other alternatives first. Then, if nothing else works, begin to entertain the thought of surgery. Surgery, while it may be necessary, is the last resort.

Straight Talk

Many years ago, I developed severe pain in my left shoulder while golfing and it became so persistent that I was incredibly limited in the use of my left arm. I became so desperate that when the doctor mentioned that surgery was an option, I jumped on it. He said that there were alternatives, but I was stubborn and thought that surgery would be the cure. Instead of an immediate cure, it became an over-nine month ordeal. What I learned was that whether or not I had the surgery, I still needed to do the rehab. When I talked with a physical therapist friend, she told me (rather emphatically) that I could have possibly received the same results in less time, if I had done the rehab route.

Most physicians I know will try every alternative before surgery. First, they may suggest an anti-inflammatory. Inflammation needs to be managed immediately, and for some people, an anti-inflammatory and rest can solve the issue, especially in the acute (beginning) stage. The next suggestion is often physical therapy. Really good physical therapists are worth their weight in gold. They can figure out what exercises are right for you, and can use other modalities like hands-on bodywork, ultrasound, and muscle stimulation to help manage your pain. If that doesn't work, your physician might suggest an epidural injection. This is the beginning of a more invasive course of treatment. Only after exhausting all of these treatments should surgery be considered. But you do need to remember that the healing process takes time and you need to allow your body that time to heal. Don't expect miracles or that your back pain will be cured overnight.

The Self-Assessment

Since you probably won't be coming through my doors here in Washington, D.C., you will perform a self-assessment to get a baseline picture of your condition before you begin. I often tell my students that if something is not measurable, it's not meaningful. You want to know from where you are starting to know how far you've come.

The self-assessment is rather easy to do. There are only three things you need: the floor, the wall, and a camera (your smartphone will work just fine). You are looking for postural deviations and muscular imbalances, which will show up in your body as something that deviates from the "norm." There is an ideal posture that we all would like to achieve and maintain. For some people, perfect posture may be an unrealistic goal, but it is worthwhile to improve ourselves so that we come closer to ideal posture. If possible, take a picture of yourself during each assessment. It will give you a great before-and-after comparison that is truly measurable; you will see the difference in the photos.

Posture Assessment

What is good posture? The Cleveland Clinic defines proper posture as "the position in which you hold your body upright against gravity while standing, sitting or lying down. Good posture involves training your body to stand, walk, sit and lie in positions where the least strain is placed on supporting muscles and ligaments during movement or weight-bearing activities."[1] You should be able to hold your body in proper alignment so that there is freedom of movement while providing the proper stability to all the joints to hold them in place. It's all about efficiency and effortless movement.

Remember when you were a kid playing with your friends? Your body just moved; you didn't think about it, it was effortless and efficient. It did what you asked of it, no more or less. It supported all the motions you wanted it to do. While twisting, turning, running, walking, climbing, and jumping, your body supported you properly. As we age, through disuse and abuse, our bodies tend to stiffen up and we lose our proper postural spinal curves. It may be that we hold too much weight or that we slouch while at our desk or while watching TV. These, along with countless other poor posture choices made over the years, have led to the posture you see in the mirror. Often, your environment is the culprit. Things such as your desk chair, the height and angle of your computer monitor, the constant use of your cell phone (looking down to text is a huge cause of poor posture), and the position of your car's seat—all of these have an effect on your posture.

About 10 years ago I was talking with a physical therapist friend and she noticed that my posture could be improved. Okay, honestly, it was downright awful. She told me to get a straight back chair for my office and home. I thought she was out of her mind. Am I never allowed to be comfortable again? This was, in my opinion, a rather drastic prescription, but I think there is a middle-of-the-road approach that can benefit all.

I suggest using a timer on your desk or computer that you can set to go off once an hour. When the alarm sounds, adjust your posture and try to maintain it for 30 seconds to a minute. Don't force it, just make gentle corrections; tuck your chin slightly, pull your head back, lift your chest a bit, and sit up taller in your seat by sitting on your "sits bones" (the bones in your butt) as you place both feet flat on the floor. After a month or so, decrease the timer's countdown to 40 minutes then eventually down to 30 minutes and so on. When it gets down to about 15 minutes, you will be surprised how much easier it is to adjust your posture. While you are decreasing your timer's countdown, you can increase the amount of time you are holding better posture. Start at 30 seconds and work up to two or three minutes. Over time, you will find that you will build endurance in these small postural muscles and it will become easier to maintain good posture for longer and longer periods of time.

Do you want another reason to improve and maintain proper posture? Remember the curves in your spine we discussed in chapter one? We want them to be gentle curves, not steep or exaggerated curves. Any exaggeration of the curves to our spine will put undue stress on the spine and the surrounding tissues. When you have these exaggerated spinal curves—increased kyphosis (thoracic) and lordosis (lumbar and cervical)—you are increasing the amount of compression force that your discs experience. Let's face it, we exhibit poor posture most of the day, so these compressive forces are fairly constant. It gets worse when we stay in one position for prolonged periods of time. I hear from many clients that they will stay at their desk for hours on end without moving. This lack of movement is terrible for your spine, which is made to move. Remember that your discs get their nutrition from movement. Proper posture, or even improved posture, will begin to take some pressure off these discs, allowing them to be properly nourished and able to move optimally.

This self-assessment requires you to have someone take two pictures of you: one from the back, and one from the side. And I am not talking about a selfie.

I want the picture to be taken from far enough away that your whole body is in the frame. I want you to be relaxed and not trying to maintain perfect posture. I want a natural stance, as this is the only way to get an accurate picture of your starting point. This is usually a reality check. Most people when taking a selfie or picture do their best to accentuate their positives and reduce their negatives. I have a friend who is self-conscious about her weight so every time she is in a picture, she stands behind other people so only her face is showing. In these self-assessment photos, no hiding. This picture is only for you, no one else. You should be dressed in something that will display your body. For women, I recommend form-fitting tights and a sports bra. For men, shorts and no shirt is usually best, or at least a form-fitting tank top or undershirt.

In your photos, look for postural issues and compare and contrast your pictures with those in figure 3.1, then answer the questions in figure 3.2. The main postural deviations are going to be:

- *Sway back.* Your ribs sit behind your hips causing increased compression on your low back. This often presents as rounded shoulders and a forward head carriage (see figure 3.1*a*).

- *Lumbar lordosis.* There is a large arch to your low back resulting in increased compression of the lumbar discs, an anterior tilt (tipping forward) of the pelvis, and tight hamstrings and hip flexors (see figure 3.1*b*).

- *Kyphosis of the thoracic spine.* This usually presents as rounded shoulders, forward head carriage, and a tucked-under pelvis (see figure 3.1*c*).

- *Flat back.* This condition is when your spine is straighter than it should be. The spinal curves have decreased leaving your cervical, thoracic, and lumbar spines flattened out. (see figure 3.1*d*).

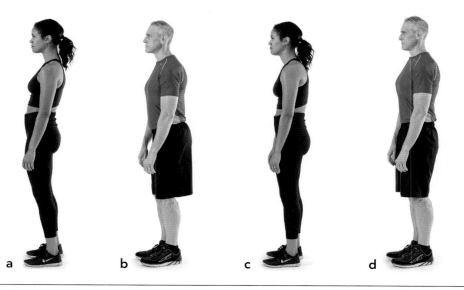

a   b   c   d

FIGURE 3.1 Main postural deviations: *(a)* sway back, *(b)* lumbar lordosis, *(c)* kyphosis of the thoracic spine, and *(d)* flat back.

Figure 3.2 Posture assessment checklist

Side

Look at the photo taken from the side. Starting with the head and working your way down, answer the following questions:

Is your head forward?	___ yes ___ no
Do you have rounded shoulders?	___ yes ___ no
Are your hands facing behind you?	___ yes ___ no
Is your rib cage behind your pelvis?	___ yes ___ no
Do you have an exaggerated curve to your low back?	___ yes ___ no
Does your belt line tip forward in the front?	___ yes ___ no
Are your knees locked out?	___ yes ___ no

Behind

Look at the photo taken from behind. Starting with the head and working your way down, answer the following questions:

Are you holding your head straight?	___ yes ___ no
Is one shoulder higher than the other?	___ yes ___ no
Are your shoulders shifted sideways over your hips?	___ yes ___ no
Is one hip higher than the other?	___ yes ___ no

From B. Richey, *Back Exercise*. (Champaign, IL: Human Kinetics, 2021).

Don't worry, everyone has some postural deviations. *Everyone.* You aren't looking for tiny deviations, you are looking for the big ones. The small ones are usually related to activities of daily life, caused by actions such as how you carry your purse, briefcase, or backpack, or if you hold your phone between your shoulder and your ear while talking. This could cause your head to tilt slightly even when you're not using your phone. If you look hard enough for something, you're bound to find it or, more accurately, create it. So, ignore the small deviations and put your focus on the obvious ones. Remember that you are using this as a starting point. When you become stronger and your back pain has diminished, you will revisit these photos and you will be able to see if there has been a change in your overall posture.

Wall Test

This self-assessment will evaluate the amount of curvature in your low back, known as lordosis. Every spine needs some curvature, but too large a curve can lead to increased compression, which places undue stress on the spine and can ultimately cause pain.

To assess this, stand with your back and heels against a wall. (For those of you who have more ample rear ends you may want to have your heels a little further from the wall.) With your hand, evaluate how much space you have between the wall and your low back, and determine where that space is located. Ideally, you should just be able to put your hand flat behind your low back (see figure 3.3). The space between the wall and your hand should be relatively small: a couple of inches or so. If you can fit your fist in this space, then you have a little too much of a lordosis. A colleague of mine, Sue Hitzmann, offers a great analogy on this topic. She says your low back should resemble the small bridge over a koi pond, not the Golden Gate Bridge. You want to have a small gentle curve to your low back.

Another facet to evaluate is the location of the curve. Some people have a low curve right behind the belly button, which is ideal. However, some often have a much higher curve that extends up into the mid-back. When doing your self-assessment, determine if your curve is behind the belly button or much higher. A higher midback curve often corresponds to tight muscles in the ribcage and thoracic region. The next self-assessment will discuss this further.

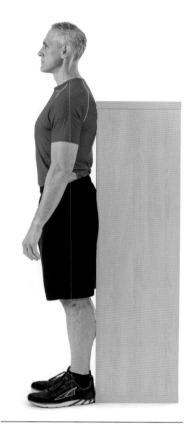

FIGURE 3.3 Evaluating lordosis using the wall test.

Lying Overhead Reach Test

The lying overhead reach test is going to evaluate the mobility of your thoracic spine and ribcage. Ideally, your thoracic spine should be able to freely extend as well as rotate. Limitations in thoracic mobility can lead to or contribute to low back pain. If you have limited movement in your thoracic spine, your lumbar spine will be asked to move beyond its capabilities, which can lead to injury. This assessment should be done on the floor; a bed is too soft and will not give you accurate results. There are two parts to this test and both are performed lying down with your feet on the floor and knees bent at 90 degrees.

For the first part of the test, place your hand under your low back as you did in the last test. Where is your arch and how big is it? Is it a small arch under your belly button? Or is it a midback arch, with the arch going up into the lower part of the ribs? Take note of its location and size.

The second part of the test begins with hands at the sides. Keeping your arms straight, lift your hands above your chest (see figure 3.4*a*), then continue moving your arms overhead until your arms are by your ears (see figure 3.4*b*). Feel what happens when your arms move from your sides to your ears. Do you feel as though your arch increased or crept up higher on your back, or did it stay low? Do you feel your ribcage lift and tilt back toward your head as your arms went overhead, or did your ribs remain stable and normal? If you felt the arch inch upward and increase, and felt your ribs "flare" out, this indicates that your ribcage and thoracic region is extremely tight and needs to be addressed.

While lying down, I also want you to notice what your head is doing. Does your head relax on the ground without a pillow? When you lie down, where do your eyes and nose point? If your eyes and nose are tilted, looking back over your head rather than straight ahead, this is another indication of thoracic tightness. When our thoracic spine is tight or fixated, more stress may be placed on the lumbar spine. Thoracic mobility will be covered in chapter 6.

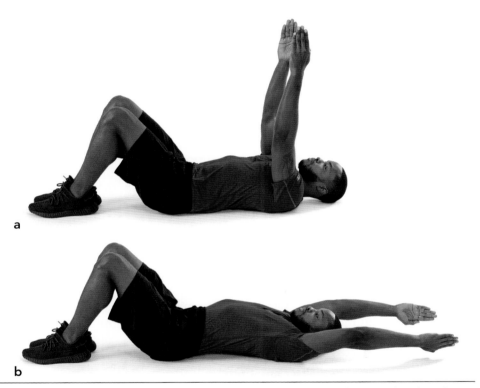

a

b

FIGURE 3.4   Evaluating the mobility in your thoracic spine with the lying overhead reach test.

Thomas Test

This self-assessment evaluates your hip flexor tightness. Tight hip flexors often go hand in hand with low back pain. The Thomas test is named after Dr. Hugh Owen Thomas, a British orthopedic surgeon who created the test to rule out hip flexion contracture.[2] Over the years, it has been commonly used to evaluate tightness in the hip flexors, quadriceps, and iliotibial bands. This is a modified version of the test that you can do yourself.

Lying on your back with your feet on the floor and knees at 90 degrees, bring one knee tightly into your chest, then bring the other knee up so that both knees are pulled to your chest (see figure 3.5a). This should flatten your back and stabilize your pelvis. It is important that during this test you don't let your back arch at all; keep it flat on the ground. Extend the bottom leg straight on the ground (see figure 3.5*b*). (If any of this causes you any low back pain, stop. There are some conditions where flattening your back may cause discomfort.)

Are you able to get your bottom leg flat on the floor? If so, then your hip flexors aren't overly tight. However, if your knee is far from able to touch the ground or your leg is suspended off the floor, then you will need to address your hip flexors. Hip flexor stretches will be included in chapter 8.

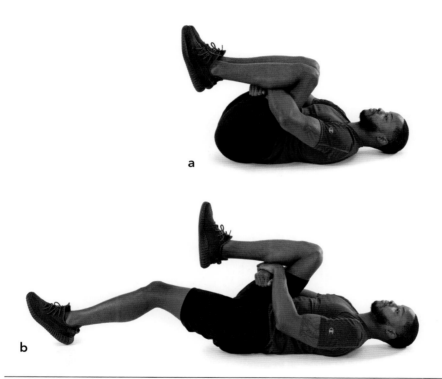

FIGURE 3.5   Evaluating hip flexor tightness with the Thomas test.

Tabletop Hold Test

This self-assessment evaluates your abdominal endurance in a static position. Abdominal or core strength is vitally important in improving low back pain.[3] You need to assess the current endurance level of these abdominal muscles to gauge your starting point. This assessment is also a great exercise in and of itself.

This self-assessment is timed. Lying on your back with your feet flat on the floor, knees at 90 degrees, bring one leg up so that your knee is directly above your hip and your knee is bent at 90 degrees. Then, bring your other leg up next to it. Your shins should be parallel to the floor, creating a "tabletop" position (see figure 3.6). Make sure your head stays down throughout the test; lifting your chin to your chest is cheating. Hold this position for as long as you can, comfortably. This should not cause any strain or pain. If it does, stop. You are not in competition with anyone; this is just to gauge a starting point.

For some people, just getting into the tabletop position may cause pain. There was a time when my back was acting up so much that simply lifting the second leg into position caused my back some discomfort, and I found myself straining slightly to keep them suspended. Don't worry if this happens to you. It is okay. Others will find that they can hold it for 30 seconds or more, and that's great. This indicates that you already possess some core strength. As you progress in the program, you will find that your core strength will increase significantly and your endurance level for this activity will increase as well.

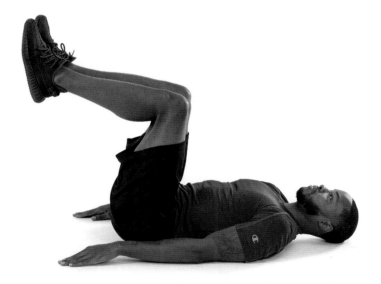

FIGURE 3.6   Evaluating abdominal endurance using the tabletop hold test.

Pain Awareness Journal

Next, I want you to keep a body awareness journal. This is nothing special that you need to buy, just use a regular composition book, notebook, or even a note taking app on your phone. I want you to be honest with yourself and evaluate your daily discomfort level. Some people hold on to their pain and it becomes a part of them that they aren't willing or ready to release. Becoming aware of how much discomfort you are in will make it easier to identify your true degree of pain, and you will begin to understand how persistent it is. It will make it easier for you to let it go.

At the beginning of your journal, I'd like you to answer a few questions, and it's okay if you don't know the answers immediately; you can always add them in as you go. The first question is "What is your pain level today?" You want a starting point, something to compare to down the road. Don't overthink this; go with the first number that pops into your head.

Second question: "What makes the pain worse?" Is there a specific motion that causes an increase in pain? I have multiple bulging or herniated discs from long ago that I continue to manage with exercise. I also know that if I am sitting down and I side bend all the way to the left, it will cause a flare-up so I tend to avoid this motion. With your pain, it may not be a single movement that causes it. Maybe it is a complex motion or series of movements. Maybe it's getting up out of a chair, rolling over in bed, walking down stairs, or taking long walks. Each of these activities indicate a different issue. If getting out of a chair increases your pain, that could indicate that your hip flexors are tight and that you have a hard time straightening up, or that your core and lower-body strength are weak and you aren't able to support yourself upon rising. Or it could tell me that you need to move around more, that sitting for too long is the culprit. So, what makes the pain worse? Remember that you can always add to this list as we go. If something happens and you realize that another motion causes pain, write that down as well.

The next question is "What makes the pain better?" Is there something that alleviates the pain? I had a college friend who injured her back badly while doing a lot of bending, squatting, and twisting in shallow water. She wasn't used to these motions, and it really caused her pain. The only place she felt comfortable and could get some relief was sitting in my old beat-up recliner. For some reason, this took all the pressure off her back and she was able to get comfortable and even sleep. Is there anything that makes you feel better? Is it sitting, laying down, or perhaps moving and exercising? Take note of what makes you feel better and relieves your pain, and determine if it helps every time. This reveals a lot about the position or positions that may be best for you. For example, perhaps you experience most of your discomfort standing, but as soon as you sit down, it goes away. Maybe flattening your back and being in a posterior pelvic tilt is better for you, at least to start. For other people, just taking pressure off the back by sitting in a recliner or comfortable chair, like my friend discovered, gives relief. Find out what, if anything, provides relief for you.

The body awareness journal is for you and you alone. There are many different ways to use it, and I want you to discover what works best for you. One approach is to record your level of pain at the end of the day. Try to remember back for the entire day and honestly rate your pain. This is the easiest and fastest way to use the journal. But there are other options.

You can be more detailed and specific. For example, say you woke up and your discomfort level was at a 2 or a 3. As you moved around, you felt better, and perhaps it decreased to a 1 or a 2. You then sat at work all day and your back tightened up; by 5 p.m. you were at a 4 or a 5. You came home and now at bedtime the pain is only at a 1. The specificity of this method is helpful because it not only keeps you honest but it also identifies patterns. What this pattern tells me is that movement seems to help. What began as stiffness when you woke up, eased a bit when you were moving around. After sitting and not moving it became worse. Then after work it eased even more. Evaluate your office set-up to make sure it is best for your body because proper ergonomics are important. I would also recommend getting up from your desk every hour and doing some easy activities to keep your body moving throughout the day.

What if you discover that you were in a lot of discomfort on Monday but felt better as the week went on, and by Friday you were doing okay; then on the following Monday you were feeling worse again? This indicates that something you're doing over the weekend could be making things worse. I've had a number of clients do hours of gardening on the weekend and never realize that all those hours of bending and twisting may be making things worse. I laugh because I've had clients blame me, claiming they are in pain because of our last workout, but a little digging reveals that they went on a very long hike or did some gardening. Their bodies may not have been prepared for these activities, causing inflammation and the true source of their pain. But at the same time, I am really happy that they felt that they could do these activities. They weren't afraid to try. Sometimes pain can make our lives very limited. Over time, as they continue to get stronger, they will be able to perform these activities without pain.

Keeping a journal allows you to become aware and to become honest with yourself about what you are truly feeling, and at the same time identifies some patterns that may help you make changes in your daily life that can affect your pain level. Over time, your overall pain level should begin to decrease until pain isn't a daily issue for you anymore. This journal is not something you write in forever, just for a while and especially at the beginning. What I notice is that people stop using their journals as they begin to feel better and don't need it anymore.

Assessment is important to do; it will be an indicator of how far you've progressed three to six months down the line. Retest yourself three months from now, and then again in another three months. You should see an improvement. Remember pain is not always the best indicator of success. As you get stronger, your pain level should reduce. However, I really want you to focus on what you are able to do. Are you able to lift, carry, walk, and move better than you did before starting the program? That is the level of success I wish for you.

PART II

Exercises

Joseph Pilates once said, "Physical fitness can neither be achieved by wishful thinking, nor outright purchase." He was absolutely correct. You might feel like you've taken a big step by purchasing this book—but if it just sits on your shelf, it's not going to make a difference. Simply reading these next chapters about exercise, without doing them, won't help your back get any better, either. So, you've bought the book, and now you're reading it: It's time for action. It's time to take the first step to managing your low back pain. It's time to move.

If you've already read the first section, you have a basic understanding of anatomy, and perhaps you jumped ahead to section three to learn about your own pathology. Now you're ready to learn the specific exercises that will help manage your condition.

Look at the first month of exercises listed in the schedule for your condition. There should be between 8 to 12 exercises. These are divided into the different stages of spinal stabilization we talked about in chapter 2. In the beginning you will spend the majority of the time working on spinal stabilization on the ground, with a little flexibility added in toward the end. As you progress, you will discover that you are doing more varied exercises that involve different positions, with the goal of gaining the ability to exercise in any position—lying, seated, or standing—with no pain.

These exercises go into great detail about form and performance to ensure you do the exercises correctly and don't risk further injury. Take your time performing the exercises and really focus on them. Many people just go through the motions and don't get everything they can out of the exercise. If you zero in and put all of your attention into each exercise, it will pay off in the end.

When you first start doing the exercises, they may take longer than expected. Don't worry. As you progress and become more efficient, you'll move through them more quickly, but don't rush. Most of my clients spend anywhere from 15 to 30 minutes doing their exercises. That's not much to ask in order to stabilize and strengthen your spine. For additional information and selected videos explaining some of the foundational and more difficult exercises, you can visit www.backexercisebook.com.

After you've completed one month, move on to the next. You will be surprised how easy the exercises are once you've done them a few times. If you feel that you want to repeat a month before moving on, please do—there is no harm in continuing to repeat the exercises for an additional month until you're really comfortable doing them. Listen to your body. Some clients believe that a certain exercise is their "holy grail" exercise, the one that makes the most difference. If you find that to be true, add it in each month if it isn't already there. Every body is different, and you need to listen to yours. Do the exercises and you will get stronger and, most importantly, more stable in your spine. A stable spine means you can build a strong body around it and reduce or eliminate your pain. Here are the exercises that will start you down the right path.

CHAPTER 4

Supine and Prone Exercises

"Out of curiosity, when will we be getting off the floor and doing some real exercise?" You wouldn't believe how many times I have been asked this question. No matter who comes into my facility, we start with "foundation exercises" that focus on building a solid foundation, and spinal stability work is the cornerstone of these exercises.

When you build a new home, the allure of spending most of your time and energy on the finishing touches is strong. All the eye candy, from appliances to paint to flooring, makes it easy to get caught up in what the house will look like when it's finished. However, it's the boring but crucial elements—the foundation under and behind the paint and finishes—that should take most of the time, effort, and budget. If you build your home on a weak foundation, it will never last. Your body is exactly the same.

We will build your body from the inside out, focusing on what's underneath rather than on the muscles you see in the mirror. Remember that the spinal stabilizers are the deepest muscles of your lumbar spine. These foundation exercises will be performed primarily in the supine position (lying on your back) and are referred to as *fully supported exercises*. Because you are lying on your back, the ground will be giving you a great deal of support. These exercises will require your full focus at the beginning. In fact, I've been told many times that this part feels more like an exercise for the brain. Find yourself a distraction-free place to perform the exercises if possible. The more attention you can give the exercises the more you will get out of them.

And returning to the question, "When will we be getting off the floor?" my answer is this: Once you master these exercises and have started to create a more stable spine, you will have earned the right to move on to the next level, partially supported spinal stability exercises, which we will cover in the next chapter.

Supine Exercises

The exercises presented here are performed in a supine position. We consider this a fully supported position because your entire backside is planted on the ground. This is the greatest amount of external support you can have during exercise.

For all these exercises, lightly engage your Kegel muscles (pelvic muscles), maintain a neutral spine (whatever your condition dictates a neutral spine to be), and focus on what is not moving—namely your spine and pelvis—rather than what is moving. All exercises will start at 10 repetitions and work up to 30 repetitions. Start with two sets and work up to three.

Engaging Your Kegel Muscles

I'm sure some of you are already aware of your Kegel muscles. But many people, especially men, haven't got a clue. In fact, it has been speculated that the Kegel muscles are the most underutilized muscles in the male anatomy.

When we talk about our Kegels, we are actually talking about the pelvic floor muscles. Imagine your pelvis is a bowl, and your pelvic floor muscles create the lining of the bowl. When these muscles contract, they pull the pelvis together, giving it internal support. If it weren't for these muscles, your insides wouldn't be inside anymore.

You want these pelvic floor muscles to be active during the exercises. They (the piriformis, coccygeus, levator ani, and perineum) attach to the pelvis and to the sacrum and coccyx, acting together to lift the floor of your pelvis, kind of like a hammock. We don't want these muscles to be so loose that they sag, nor do we want them to be too tight. (If contracting these muscles creates discomfort, please talk to your doctor.) They attach to the lowest part of your spine so they are important muscles to learn to engage during exercise.

How do you engage your Kegel? To describe how to locate the Kegel muscles, it's necessary to be somewhat graphic. For women, the easiest way to feel the Kegel is to imagine squeezing the walls of the vagina around a tampon. These are the muscles that need to fire. For men, the best way to feel these muscles contract is to imagine drawing the testicles up off the floor into your pelvis, or imagine holding back a stream of urine.

Now that you have located these muscles, it is important to note that you do not need to hold them extremely tight. In fact, the opposite is true. Engage them at about 30 percent of a maximum squeeze. In other words, it should be a light hold. Again, I use the analogy of a baby bird. Imagine you are holding a baby bird. You want to hold it firm enough so that it doesn't fly away but not so tight that you hurt it. A light hold is all that is necessary. This should be held throughout the exercises.

Bent-Knee Fallout

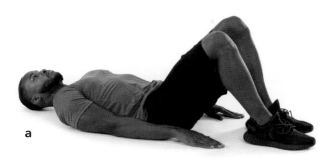

a

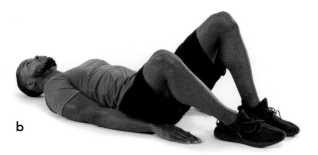

b

Objective

To create spinal stability while moving the hips. Keep the pelvis level and stable, not allowing it to twist from side to side.

Starting Position

Lie on the back with the knees bent at 90 degrees and feet flat on the floor (a). You can place the hands on the hip bones as a feedback device.

Movement

Slowly drop one knee out to the side and toward the ground, more slowly than you think you should (b). Let the foot rotate with the knee; it doesn't need to stay flat on the floor. Most people only get to about 30 degrees to 45 degrees before their pelvis begins to move. That is where to stop, then slowly bring the knee back up to the starting position and repeat with the other side. How far the knee travels doesn't matter for now. Over time, you will gain a greater range of motion while keeping the spine still. You know you are going slow enough when there is some "chattering" in the leg muscles. This is a good thing. This means that the smaller muscles of the pelvis are firing. If you go too fast, you will bypass these smaller (stabilizing) muscles and only use the larger (mobilizing) muscles.

Heel Slide

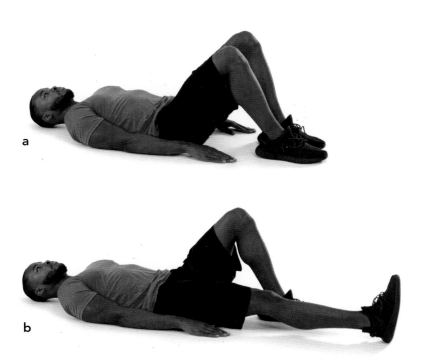

a

b

Objective

To create spinal stability while extending the legs. Keep the pelvis level so that it does not tilt while extending the legs. Do not arch or flatten the back at all during this exercise. Maintain a neutral spine.

Starting Position

Lie on the back with the knees bent at 90 degrees and feet flat on the floor (a). This exercise is best done on a surface where the feet will slide.

Movement

Slowly extend one leg forward by sliding the heel along the surface as far as possible without losing a neutral spine (b). The foot doesn't need to stay flat on the surface; only the heel needs to remain in contact. You may be able to extend all the way or only get halfway, and that's okay. When you've gone as far as possible without changing the spinal angle, return to the starting position and repeat on the other side.

Marching

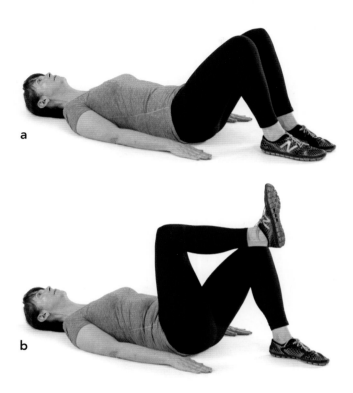

a

b

Objective
To create spinal stability while lifting the legs. Maintain a stable spine to keep the pelvis from twisting or tipping forward or back. Don't let the pelvis tuck, tilt, or twist.

Starting Position
Lie on the back with the knees bent at 90 degrees and the feet flat on the floor (*a*).

Movement
Lift one knee so the thigh is perpendicular to the ground (*b*). Return the leg to the ground and repeat on the other side. While this seems easy enough, in all my years I have only had a couple of people do it correctly the first time. On the next repetition, be conscious about what the resting leg is doing. It should be resting, yet most people tend to push down with that leg to use the leg muscles to stabilize the pelvis and spine rather than using the core. I want you to focus on keeping the resting leg relaxed and make sure it does not push down as you lift the active leg. If you do it correctly, you should feel additional engagement of your abdominal (core) muscles. You will alternate legs, each time relaxing one leg while engaging the other.

March-Up

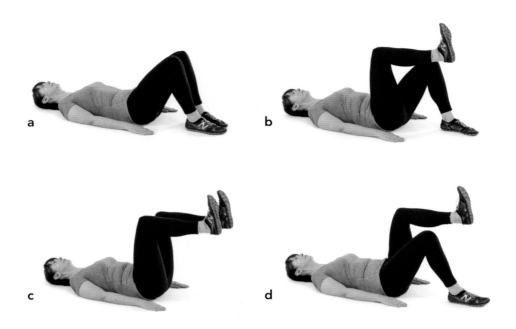

Objective
To keep the spine stable as you bring the legs up into a tabletop position and back down. Do not let the back arch or flatten, and maintain a neutral spine throughout the exercise.

Starting Position
Lie on the back with the knees bent at 90 degrees and the feet flat on the floor (*a*).

Movement
Draw the right knee up until the leg is in a tabletop position (*b*). Stabilize the pelvis, engage the core, and lift the left leg so that both legs are now in tabletop position (*c*). Hold briefly, then lower the right leg and then the left (*d*). On the next repetition, start by lifting the left leg followed by the right leg, then lower the left leg, followed by the right leg. Continue alternating starting legs.

Leg Lowering

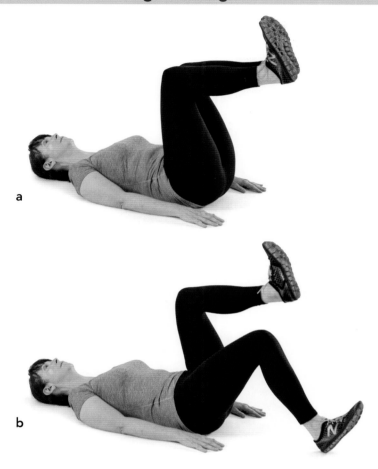

a

b

Objective
To keep the spine stable as you lower the legs. Keep the knees over the navel without letting them float further away toward the chest. Maintain a neutral spine throughout the exercise.

Starting Position
Lie on the back with the knees bent at 90 degrees and the feet flat on the floor. Lift one leg into a tabletop position, followed by the other leg and then hold the tabletop position (a).

Movement
Slowly lower one leg until the foot taps down on the floor or the back arches, whichever comes first (b). If you feel the back begin to arch, that is as far as you go. Lift the leg back up to the tabletop position and repeat with the opposite leg, lowering it toward the ground and then lifting it back up to tabletop position. Make sure to lower one foot to the floor at a time; if you drop both at the same time you have a greater likelihood of straining the low back.

Advanced Kick-Out

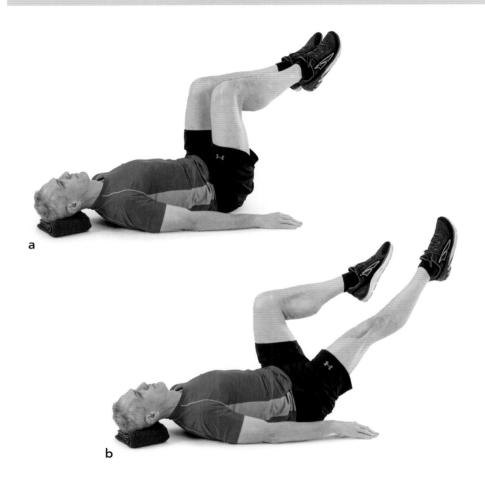

a

b

Objective
To maintain a neutral spine as you kick out the leg. Do not let the back arch or flatten.

Starting Position
Lie on the back with the knees bent at 90 degrees and the feet flat on the floor. Lift one leg into a tabletop position, followed by the other leg, and then hold the tabletop position (a).

Movement
Kick one foot out into the air at a 45-degree angle (b) and return to the starting position, then repeat with the other leg. Make sure the back doesn't arch during the kick. If it does, aim the foot higher rather than down toward the ground. This shortens the lever of the leg and makes the exercise a little easier. Make sure to stabilize the pelvis between each repetition.

Dying Bug

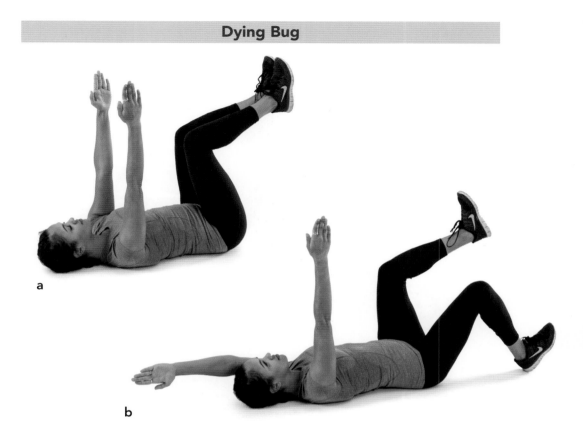

a

b

Objective

To combine upper- and lower-body movement while keeping the spine stable. Maintain a neutral spine throughout the exercise.

Starting Position

Lie on the back with the knees bent at 90 degrees and the feet flat on the floor. Lift one leg into a tabletop position, followed by the other leg, and then hold the tabletop position. Bring the arms to a position in front of the chest (*a*).

Movement

Lower one foot to the ground while at the same time extending the opposite arm back over the head (*b*). Return both the arm and leg to the starting position, then repeat with the opposite arm and leg. Because there is a high amount of coordination involved with this exercise, you may make contact between the hand and the knee that stay at the starting position. This will make the exercise a little easier and create more abdominal engagement. As one arm and leg extend out, the opposite hand will touch the opposite knee and apply a little bit of pressure.

Clamshell

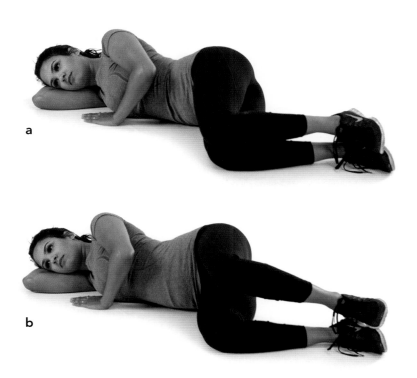

a

b

Objective
To keep the spine still while lying on the side and moving the hips. This exercise will also begin to wake up and strengthen the gluteus medius.

Starting Position
Lie on the side with the knees at 90 degrees, the hips at approximately 45 degrees, and the feet stacked on top of one another. Roll the hips slightly forward so that the top knee is slightly in front of the bottom knee (a). This will help to lock the hips in place and limit the amount of roll-back.

Movement
Keeping the hips still, lift the top knee while keeping the feet together (b). After returning to the starting position, repeat the exercise on the other side of the body. Don't worry if the knee doesn't come up very high; this is normal. The important part of this exercise is that the hips don't roll back. They must stay perfectly still while lifting and lowering the leg.

Lying Overhead Reach

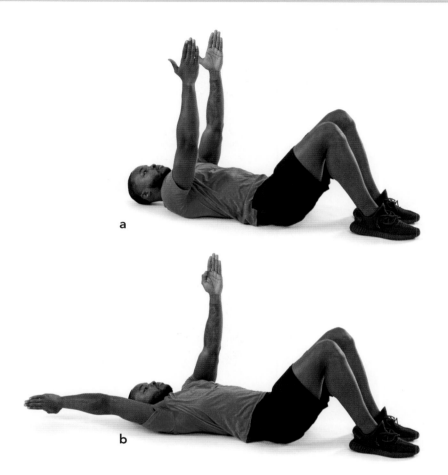

a

b

Objective
To move the arms overhead without arching the back. Make sure to do only what is achievable without arching the back. The reach of the extension isn't as important as maintaining a neutral spine throughout the exercise.

Starting Position
Lie on the back with the spine in a neutral position and the arms straight out in front of the chest (think of a zombie from a 1950s movie) (a).

Movement
While keeping the spine neutral, slowly move one arm (or both if doing a double version) back over the head without arching the back (b). Return the arm to the starting position and repeat with the other arm.

Straight-Back Bridge

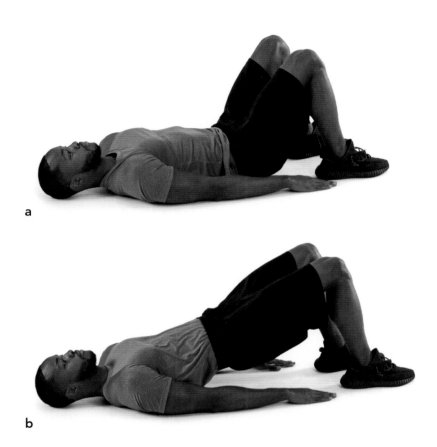

a

b

Objective
To keep the spine stable while extending from the hips. This exercise will also activate and strengthen the gluteus maximus.

Starting Position
Lie on the back with the knees bent at 90 degrees and the feet flat on the floor (a).

Movement
While maintaining a neutral spine, press down with the heels and lift the hips off the ground (b). Too often, people lift too high and end up arching the back, causing undue compression in the lumbar spine. Instead, do not go up too high, do not arch the back, and maintain a neutral spine throughout this exercise. Return the hips to the ground and repeat.

Togu Pelvic Tilt

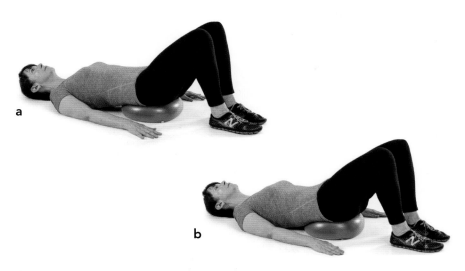

a

b

Objective
To help the pelvis move freely and to help the lower back become more flexible and supple.

Equipment
Togu ball, only slightly inflated; two to four breaths are usually enough. (If you don't have a Togu ball, you can use a mostly deflated beachball.) I recommend the Togu Pilates balance ball in a 12 inch (30 cm) size.

Starting Position
Lie on the back with the knees at 90 degrees and the feet flat on the floor. The Togu ball is placed under the sacrum (below the low back; it should not be directly on the low back) (a). Being under the sacrum will allow more freedom of movement in the pelvis, making the exercise easier and more effective than lying on the ground.

Movement
Using primarily the abdominals, perform a posterior pelvic tilt (b). If you are un- sure of what that means, imagine a neutral pelvis as a clockface with 12 o'clock being between the legs and 6 o'clock being at the navel. At the center of the clock (where the hands of the clock would rotate around) is a marble. Tilt the clock (pelvis) so that marble moves toward 6 o'clock. Then return to the start (marble back to the center). Do not tilt the clock the opposite way, which would cause the back to arch. Remember to use the abs to perform this exercise and not the legs.

Variation
For an advanced version of this exercise, perform the exercise as described, but do so with your legs up in a tabletop position. The focus should be on reaching upward, with the knees toward the sky instead of bringing the knees into the chest; this is not a rocking exercise.

Togu Marching

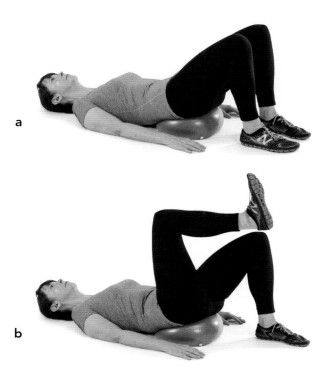

Objective
To maintain a posterior tilt in the pelvis while performing the exercise. Focus on maintaining the posterior tilt especially when the leg is returned to the floor, which is when the back will want to arch and the posterior tilt can easily be lost.

Equipment
Togu ball, only slightly inflated; two to four breaths are usually enough. (If you don't have a Togu ball, you can use a mostly deflated beachball.)

Starting Position
Lie on the back with the knees at 90 degrees and the feet flat on the floor. The Togu ball is placed under the sacrum (below the low back; it should not be directly on the low back) (a). Being under the sacrum will allow more freedom of movement in the pelvis, making the exercise easier and more effective than lying on the ground.

Movement
Using the abdominals, tilt the pelvis into a posterior position and flatten out the back and hold (refer to Togu Pelvic Tilt on page 65 for a detailed description of how to perform a posterior tilt). Lift one knee so the thigh is perpendicular to the ground (b). Return the leg to the starting position and repeat with the other leg.

Togu Tilted March-Up

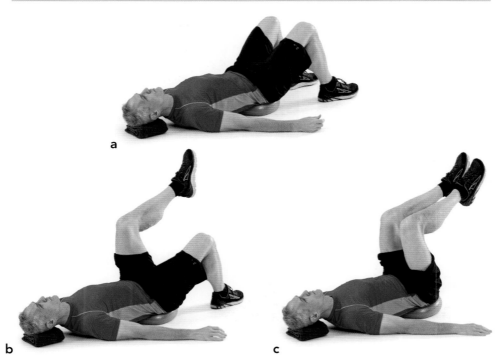

a

b   c

Objective
To maintain a posterior tilt in the pelvis while performing the exercise. Focus on maintaining the posterior tilt especially when the leg is returned to the floor, which is when the back will want to arch and the posterior tilt can easily be lost.

Equipment
Togu ball, only slightly inflated; two to four breaths are usually enough. (If you don't have a Togu ball, you can use a mostly deflated beachball.)

Starting Position
Lie on the back with the knees at 90 degrees and the feet flat on the floor. The Togu ball is placed under the sacrum (below the low back; it should not be directly on the low back) (a). Being under the sacrum will allow more freedom of movement in the pelvis, making the exercise easier and more effective than lying on the ground.

Movement
Using the abdominals, tilt the pelvis into a posterior position and flatten out the back and hold (refer to Togu Pelvic Tilt on page 65 for a detailed description of how to perform a posterior tilt). Draw the left knee up until the leg is in a table-top position (b). Stabilize the pelvis, engage the core, and lift the right leg so that both legs are now in tabletop position (c). Hold briefly, then lower the left leg and then the right. On the next repetition, start by lifting the left leg followed by the right leg, then lower the left leg followed by the right leg. Continue alternating starting legs.

Togu Leg Lowering With Pelvic Tilt

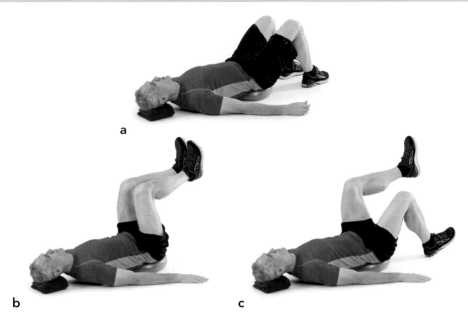

a

b   c

Objective

To maintain a posterior tilt in the pelvis while performing the exercise. Focus on maintaining the posterior tilt especially when the leg is returned to the floor, which is when the back will want to arch and the posterior tilt can easily be lost.

Equipment

Togu ball, only slightly inflated; two to four breaths are usually enough. (If you don't have a Togu ball, you can use a mostly deflated beachball.)

Starting Position

Lie on the back with the knees at 90 degrees and the feet flat on the floor. The Togu ball is placed under the sacrum (below the low back; it should not be directly on the low back) (a). Being under the sacrum will allow more freedom of movement in the pelvis, making the exercise easier and more effective than lying on the ground.

Movement

Using the abdominals, tilt the pelvis into a posterior position and flatten out the back and hold (refer to Togu Pelvic Tilt on page 65 for a detailed description of how to perform a posterior tilt). Draw the right knee up until the leg is in a tabletop position. Stabilize the pelvis, engage the core, and lift the left leg so that both legs are now in tabletop position (b). Slowly lower one leg until the foot taps down on the floor or the low back begins to arch, whichever comes first (c). The moment the low back begins to arch is your ending point. Lift the leg back up to the tabletop position and repeat with the opposite leg, lowering it toward the ground and then lifting it back up to tabletop position. Make sure to lower one foot to the floor at a time; dropping both at the same time creates a greater likelihood of low back strain.

Articulating Bridge With Togu Ball Squeeze

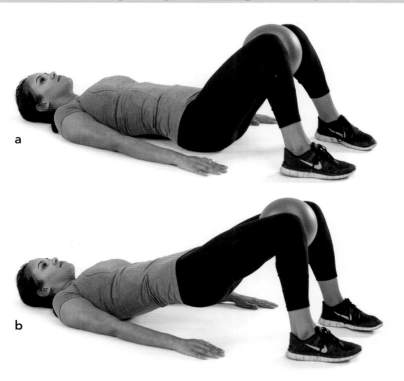

Objective
To lift the hips off the ground into a bridge using the abdominals and curling the spine to enhance spine flexibility.

Equipment
Togu ball; mostly inflated. (If you don't have a Togu ball, you can use a mostly inflated beachball.)

Starting Position
Lie on the back with the knees at 90 degrees and the Togu ball between the thighs (a). The feet are flat on the floor, slightly wider than hip-width and turned slightly inward. Pressure should be focused on the big toe rather than the outside of the foot.

Movement
Using the abdominals, move the pelvis into a posterior tilt and slowly peel the hips and spine off the floor one vertebra at a time (b). Do not go up too high and do not arch the back. You should feel a stretch in the lumbar spine at the apex of the position. Return to the starting position by trying to put the spine back down one vertebra at a time. Imagine lifting and placing a string of pearls down on a table one pearl at a time.

Prone Exercises

The exercises presented here are performed in a prone position on your stomach; the focus is on posture and the upper back muscles. This position is still considered fully supported because the entire anterior portion of the body is in contact with the ground. To avoid turning your head and altering your neck posture, use a small pillow or rolled-up towel under your forehead so your nose isn't squished against the floor. Also, remember the importance of posture to take stress off your lumbar spine. For all of these exercises, you will be lying on your stomach and pressing your pelvis into the ground to anchor your pelvis and low back.

Pelvic Press Hold

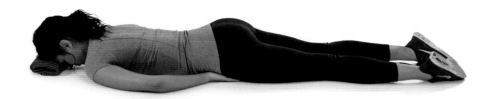

Objective
To engage the glutes and take pressure off the low back. You will perform this preparatory exercise and hold it during the remaining prone exercises for posture in this section.

Starting Position
Lie on the stomach with the forehead on a rolled-up towel or pillow, and place the hands under the pelvis just below the hip bone in the front of the body. The hands are a feedback device to make sure to push down evenly on both sides.

Movement
Press the pelvis into the hands. Hold for five seconds and release. You should feel the glutes tighten during the hold. This pelvic press will be the starting position for the next four exercises.

Pelvic Press Hip Extension

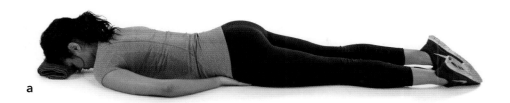

a

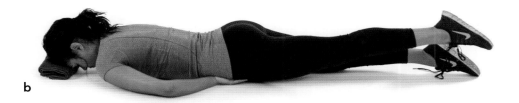

b

Objective
To perform hip extension (lifting the leg up in the air) by engaging the glutes and not engaging the low back. The goal is to only use the glutes; you should not feel the low back arch or tighten. If you do, you are lifting too high.

Starting Position
Lie on the stomach with the forehead on a rolled-up towel or pillow, and place the hands under the pelvis and press into the hands (refer to Pelvic Press Hold on page 70 for a detailed description) (a). As you press the pelvis into the hands, make sure the pressure is equal between the hands throughout the exercise.

Movement
Using the glutes, lift one leg slightly off the ground, ensuring that the pelvic pressure stays even between the hands (b). After the lifted leg returns to the ground, repeat the exercise with the other leg. This is a very difficult exercise to do correctly. Most people will twist slightly from side to side or arch the back making the pressure change as the body rocks more toward one hand and then to the other. You need to make sure to limit the range of motion and only go as high as possible while keeping the pressure even between the two sides. Even if you only lift a quarter of an inch, this is okay. Keeping the pressure even is more important than how high the leg is lifted.

Variation
With arms outstretched overhead and while performing the hip extension, add an opposite-arm lift. This is an advanced exercise and should only be done if you can perform the hip extension without arching you back.

Pelvic Press Shoulder Retraction

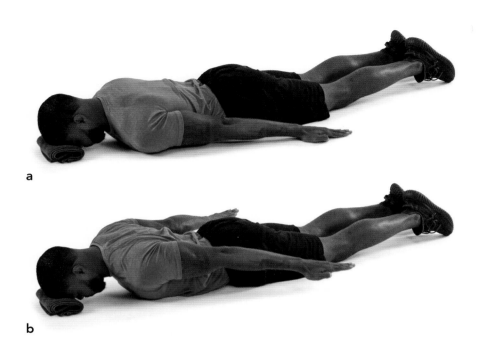

a

b

Objective

To focus on the muscles of the posterior shoulder girdle. These muscles are responsible for good posture.

Starting Position

Lie on the stomach with the forehead on a rolled-up towel or pillow and the arms at the sides with the palms facing down (a). Press the pelvis into the floor and hold (refer to Pelvic Press Hold on page 70 for a detailed description).

Movement

Pull the shoulder blades back and together; squeeze them tight and hold. Then lift the hands off the ground an inch or two (b). The lift does not have to be high; the hands only need to be slightly off the ground. Hold for 5 seconds and then relax. Work up to 10-second holds.

Pelvic Press W

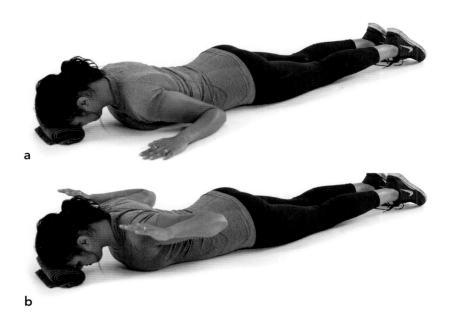

a

b

Objective

To work the muscles of the posterior shoulder girdle and rotator cuff. These muscles begin to atrophy and weaken with age and disuse so it is important to strengthen them while we are working on posture.

Starting Position

Lie on the stomach with the forehead on a rolled-up towel or pillow and the arms at the sides with the palms facing down. Press the pelvis into the floor and hold (refer to Pelvic Press Hold on page 70 for a detailed description). Move the arms into the shape of a W with the body as the center post, elbows bent with the palms just outside of the shoulders and the upper arms near the ribs (a).

Movement

Squeeze the shoulder blades together and lift the arms, with the intention of lifting the wrists higher than the elbows with the palms facing outward and pinkies higher than the thumbs (b). Hold this position for 5 seconds and then relax. Work up to 10-second holds.

Pelvic Press T

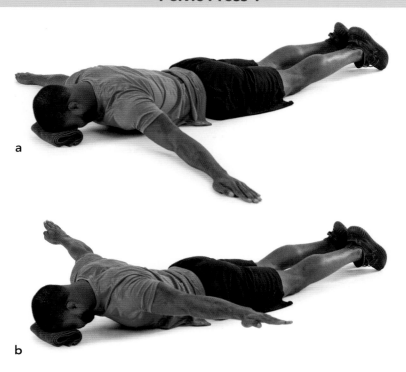

a

b

Objective
To strengthen the posterior shoulder girdle and the back of the shoulders.

Starting Position
Lie on the stomach with the forehead on a rolled-up towel or pillow and the arms at the sides with the palms facing down. Press the pelvis into the floor and hold (refer to Pelvic Press Hold on page 70 for a detailed description). Move the arms straight out from the shoulders, making a T shape (a).

Movement
Bring the shoulder blades together, then lift the arms off the ground a few inches (b). The height of the arms isn't significant, but the quality of the squeezing of the shoulder blades is crucial. Hold the contraction for 5 seconds then relax. Work up to 10-second holds.

These spinal stability exercises will create a strong foundation; everything depends on how strong of a foundation we build at the beginning of the program. These may not be exciting exercises but they will require focus and discipline. Do yourself a favor and create a distraction-free environment if possible. If your attention is drawn in too many directions, it will be difficult to perform the exercises correctly. Now that we have gone over the fully supported exercises, we are able to move on to the partially supported, unsupported, and dynamic exercises.

CHAPTER 5

Quadruped, Seated, and Standing Exercises

The previous chapter provided fully supported spinal stability exercises. This chapter discusses the next progressions in which you move your body through partially supported, unsupported, and dynamic movements while continuing to focus on keeping a stable spine throughout.

Many medical professionals agree with me that it is fairly easy to engage the core and spinal stabilizers in the supine position, but as soon as that position changes, it often feels like starting over. The supine position is the easiest position in which to control, feel, and isolate the working muscles. One reason is that you get a great amount of feedback from the ground. As soon as you move to a seated or standing position, you no longer have that support and you have to figure out how to control these muscles all over again.

The specific exercise programming in later chapters describe how, after the first month, you slowly start to include partially supported exercises, depending on your condition. Each successive month thereafter, you add more challenging exercises in various positions, all the while revisiting exercises from the positions you've already been working. We live our lives in a multitude of positions and activities, and it's vitally important to train the body in the same way. This way the strength you build will be transferable to activities of daily life and to leisure activities you enjoy.

Quadruped Exercises

The exercises presented here will be performed in the quadruped (on all fours) and in a plank position. These exercises are considered partially supported because you are still in contact with the ground at multiple points. For some of the exercises you will reduce the amount of ground contact to challenge your core stability.

Quadruped Hold

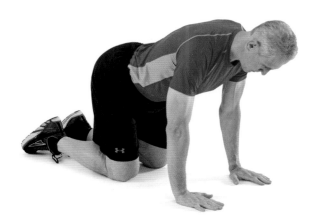

Objective
To learn how to hold the quadruped position for a length of time. This is important because developing the endurance to hold this position is necessary for completing the rest of the exercises in this section.

Starting Position
Simply holding the quadruped position can be a challenge for some, so this is a good place to start. The proper quadruped position is on the hands and knees, with the knees directly under the hips and the hands directly under the shoulders. The shoulders should be relaxed and neutral. The head is in line with the spine and not hanging down.

Movement
To find a neutral position in the shoulders, round the shoulders pushing the hands away from the chest as far as possible. Let the chest fall toward the floor bringing the shoulder blades closer together. Now, find the point that's right in the middle and usually the most comfortable. Think about keeping the shoulders away from the ears. The shoulders should be relaxed and stable at the same time. They should be stable enough that if you were pushed slightly from side to side or forward and back, you would be able to remain in the same position.

Quadruped Hold With Opposite-Arm Tap

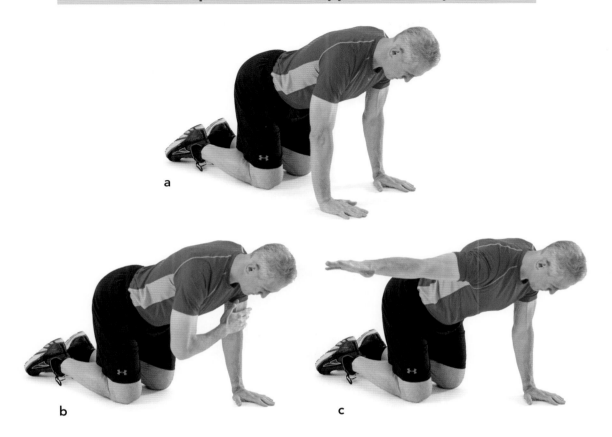

a

b

c

Objective
To force the spinal muscles to stabilize with less assistance by removing some of the points of contact.

Starting Position
Assume a quadruped position with a neutral spine (refer to Quadruped Hold on page 76 for a detailed description of this position) (a). Keep the torso as stable as possible.

Movement
While maintaining the quadruped position, take the right hand and tap the left forearm (b). Return to the quadruped starting position and repeat with the other arm. To give yourself an additional challenge, instead of tapping the opposite arm, extend your arm out to the side (c). As you lift the arm, do not let the chest fall and do not sway from side to side. This exercise is not about the tapping of the arm as much as it is about maintaining the stability of the quadruped position.

Quadruped Hip Extension Slide

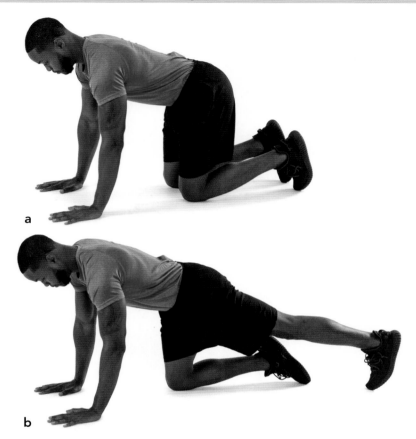

a

b

Objective

To maintain a neutral spine while moving into the leg into extension. The core needs to be engaged so the lumbar muscles aren't used to assist; only the glutes should be working to extend the leg.

Starting Position

Assume a quadruped position with a neutral spine (refer to Quadruped Hold on page 76 for a detailed description of this position) (a). Keep the torso as stable as possible.

Movement

While maintaining the quadruped position, slide one leg straight out behind the body (b). Return the leg to the starting position and continue for a specific number of repetitions before performing the exercise on the other leg. The foot position isn't important; pull the toes back toward the knee or point the toes, whichever is most comfortable. As the leg extends, keep the hips stable and do not let them slide out to the opposite side. Do not allow the lumbar muscles to do the work; do not arch the back.

Quadruped Hip Extension Lift

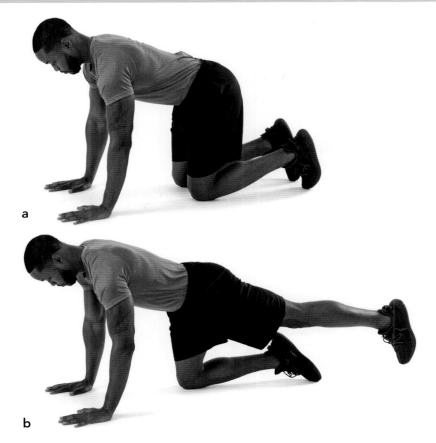

a

b

Objective
To focus on the gluteus maximus while maintaining a neutral spine in the quadruped position.

Starting Position
Assume a quadruped position with a neutral spine like the beginning of the quadruped hip extension slide (refer to Quadruped Hold on page 76 for a detailed description of this position) (a). Keep the torso as stable as possible.

Movement
Extend and lift one leg, squeezing the glutes during the lift (b). The quality of this contraction is far more important than the height of the leg lift. Only lift the leg as high as you can while keeping a neutral spine and not twisting or shifting the hips. It is normal for this to be a small range of motion so do not expect to lift the leg parallel to the ground when first starting this exercise. Lifting too high will often lead to the back wanting to arch. Return the leg to the starting position and continue for a specific number of repetitions before performing the exercise on the other leg.

Quadruped Birddog

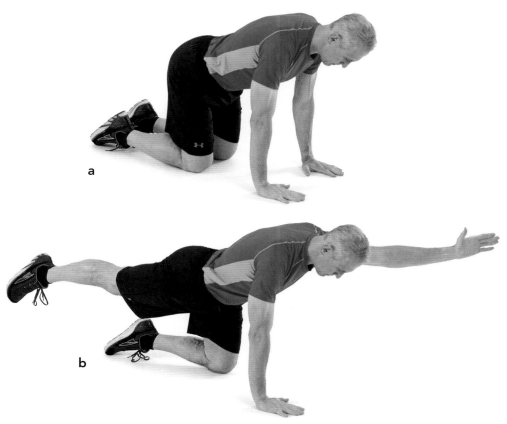

a

b

Objective
To further challenge the spinal stabilizers by removing some points of contact, and engage your spinal erectors, gluteus medius, and gluteus maximus.

Starting Position
Assume a quadruped position with a neutral spine (refer to Quadruped Hold on page 76 for a detailed description of this position) (a). Keep the torso as stable as possible.

Movement
Lift one arm straight out in front of the body while extending the opposite leg straight out behind (b). This is a fairly difficult balance challenge for most people. If you aren't able to maintain a good quadruped position, first extend the leg and then stabilize. When feeling stable, extend the opposite arm out. Hold the position for one second, then return to the quadruped starting position before switching to lift the opposite arm and leg. Work your way up to five-second holds. Remember that the range of motion isn't as important as maintaining stability. Don't let the back arch or the hips twist or sway toward the opposite direction.

High Plank

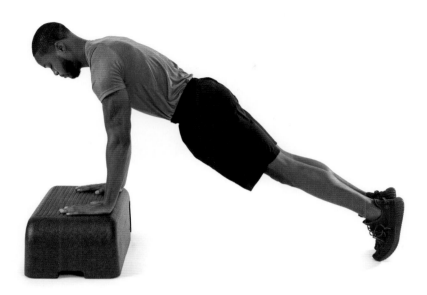

Objective
To engage the core musculature while maintaining a neutral spine.

Starting Position
Assume a push-up position with arms on a step or bench. You can also perform this exercise leaning against a wall or countertop, or with your forearms on a bed; you won't be doing the exercise with your full body weight. There should be a straight line through the ears, shoulders, ribs, hips, knees, and ankles.

Movement
Maintain the plank position as long as possible without piking the hips up in the air or letting them drop (see figure for an example using a step). This may seem like an easy exercise but many people do it incorrectly. The body needs to be in a straight line. Hold this position for 10 seconds, and work up to 30-second holds.

Full Plank

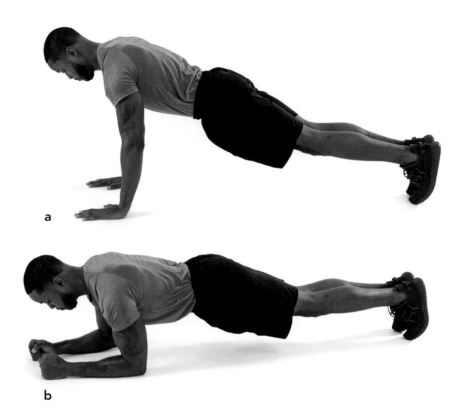

a

b

Objective
To further challenge the core and spinal stabilizers by increasing the amount of effort required to maintain the position.

Starting Position
Assume a full push-up position on the floor with the hands on the ground and the knees and hips raised (a). You shouldn't be straining to maintain this position. This can be done with the forearms on the ground to make the exercise easier (b).

Movement
Maintain the plank position as long as possible without piking the hips up in the air or letting them drop. Hold this position for 10 seconds, then lower the knees to the ground and take pressure off the body for three seconds before starting the next repetition.

Side Plank

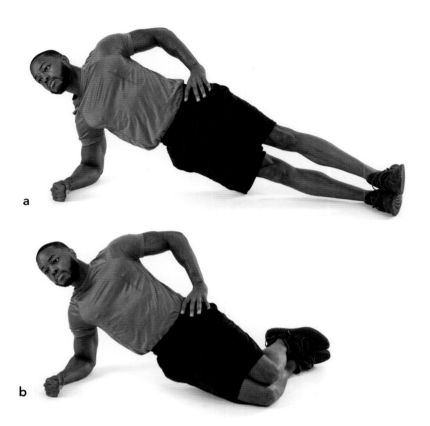

a

b

Objective
To challenge the lateral core and spinal stabilizers.

Starting Position
Begin in a side-lying position with one elbow and forearm on the ground. Lift your hips off the ground, creating a straight line between your feet and your head (a). You shouldn't be straining to maintain this position. This can also be done on your knees to make the exercise easier (b).

Movement
Maintain the side plank position as long as possible without piking the hips up in the air or letting them drop. Hold this position for 15-30 seconds, then lower the hips to rest. Then repeat the exercise on the other side.

Seated Exercises

These exercises can be done in a chair or on a stability ball for an extra challenge. They are the bridge between partially supported and unsupported positions. In a chair, these exercises would be considered partially supported because the chair is providing support, especially if you use the chair back, although I challenge you to lean forward and not rely on the chair back whenever possible. Remember that while sitting in the chair, you stabilize from the pelvis upward (the lumbar, torso, head, neck, and upper extremities) and you won't need to stabilize the lower body at all, because the chair does this for you. If performing the exercises on a stability ball, you are forced to stabilize the entire body while on the ball.

While all of the seated exercises can be done on a chair *or* a stability ball, there are some exercises included in this section that specifically require the use of a stability ball. Before you begin, make sure you have a good quality stability ball. The less expensive ones are less expensive for a reason, and the savings may cost you an injury: They aren't well made and you will have to replace them. In terms of size, if you are below five feet six inches (165 cm), use a 55 cm ball; if you are between five feet six inches (168 cm) and six feet two inches (188 cm), use the 65 cm ball; and if you are above six feet two inches (188 cm), use the 75 cm ball. I recommend the Spri Elite Xercise Ball or Balanced Body Deluxe Fitness Ball.

Also, if you have never used a stability ball, please take it easy and be careful. This is a very unstable apparatus and it can take some getting used to. Before attempting any exercise, I want you to sit on the ball and get comfortable because proper positioning is important. Your knees and hips should be at, or close to, 90 degrees. You should be able to maintain good posture on the ball, sitting tall. If you are sitting too low, the ball needs more air, and if you are sitting too high, then less air is needed. Once you are seated and relatively comfortable, move your arms around a little and see how that affects your balance and stability. As you move your arms you are creating subtle but noticeable changes in your center of gravity that will challenge the core. Once you can do that comfortably, you are ready for the exercises.

Seated Knee Lift

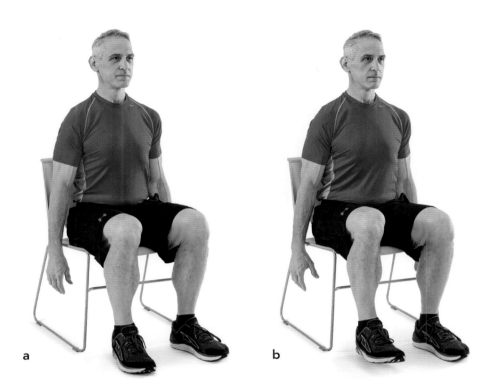

a   b

Objective
To challenge core stability and balance.

Starting Position
Sit tall in a chair, maintaining a neutral spine with arms relaxed down by the sides (a).

Movement
Lift one heel off the ground, keeping the toes on the ground. Once comfortable, lift the entire foot off the ground (b). Hold each position for a moment and then repeat with the other foot. You can add assistance by holding onto the sides of the chair for some support.

Seated Side Bend

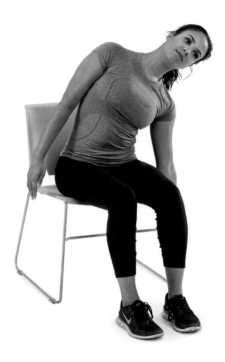

Objective
To engage the obliques as well as the quadratus lumborum and spinal erectors while still activating the spinal stabilizers during the act of side bending.

Starting Position
Sit tall in a chair with the hands at the sides and the fingers reaching toward the floor.

Movement
Gently side bend while reaching the fingers of one hand toward the ground. Return to the starting position and repeat on the other side, alternating each time. Begin with a small range of motion and slowly increase as the movement becomes comfortable.

Stability Ball Seated Hip Shift

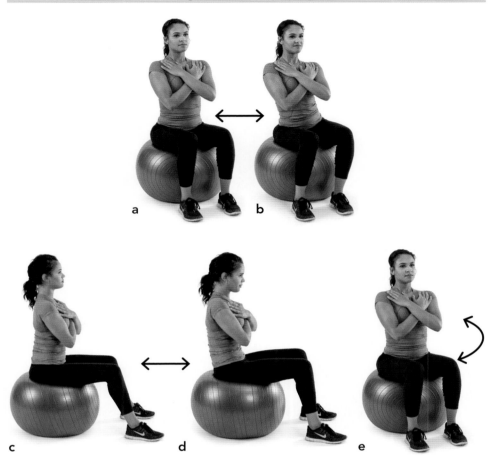

Objective
To activate the spinal stabilizers while beginning to work on slight spinal movement.

Equipment
Stability ball

Starting Position
Sit tall on the stability ball with the hands relaxed at the sides or gently on the ball if support is needed.

Movement
There are three parts to this exercise, each requiring a different movement. For each, focus on the work coming from the abdominals, not the legs. First, shift the hips from side to side (a and b). Start with a small range of motion and then increase to what feels comfortable. Next, shift the hips forward and back, tucking and tilting the pelvis (c and d). Finally, circle the hips (e).

Stability Ball Seated Knee Lift

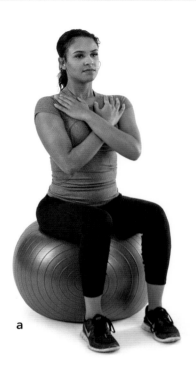

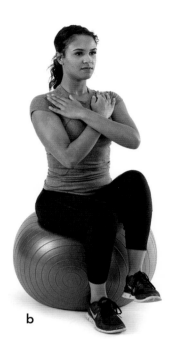

a

b

Objective
To activate the core and spinal stabilizers, and work on seated balance.

Equipment
Stability ball

Starting Position
Sit tall on the stability ball with the arms crossed at the chest (*a*).

Movement
First, lift one heel off the ground, keeping the toes on the ground. Once comfortable with this, lift the entire foot off the ground (*b*). Hold each for a moment and then alternate sides. To reduce difficulty, sit with your hands at the sides gently holding onto the ball.

Stability Ball Walk-Out

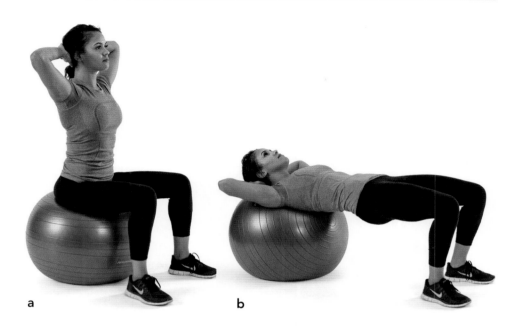

a   b

Objective
To focus on engaging the core, lower extremities, and spinal stabilizers.

Equipment
Stability ball

Starting Position
Sit tall on the stability ball with the hands behind the head or across the chest (a).

Movement
Walk the feet forward using the abs while curling the spine so that the ball slowly rolls up until it is under the upper back, as if to do crunches on the ball (b). Then, using the abdominals, curl the body back up while walking the feet back to the starting position. This is an advanced maneuver so go slowly.

Stability Ball Hip Extension Hold

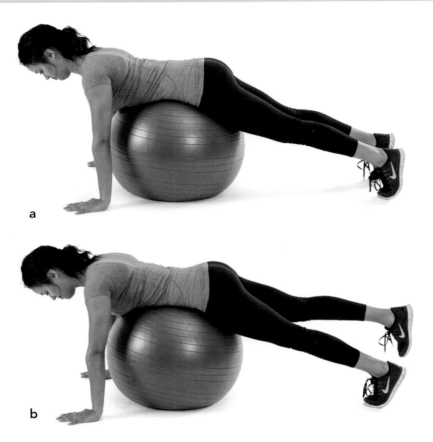

a

b

Objective
To activate and engage the gluteus maximus muscles while maintaining a neutral spine.

Equipment
Stability ball

Starting Position
Lie face down on the stability ball with the ball under the stomach and hips (a). The hands are on the ground with the arms extended and the feet are on the ground. Press the hips slightly into the ball to stabilize the hips and spine and keep the abdominals engaged (as though to lift the abs inward and away from the ball).

Movement
Lift the right leg off the ground by squeezing the right glute (b). Hold for five seconds and work up to 10-second holds. Continue for a specific number of repetitions before performing the exercise on the other leg. It is vitally important to keep the back in a neutral position throughout this exercise; do not arch the back.

Ball Birddog

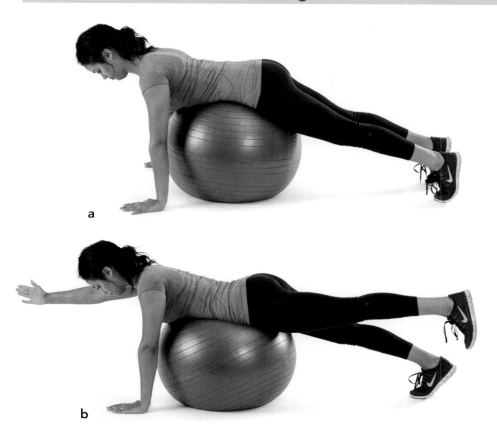

a

b

Objective
To activate the spinal stabilizers and entire posterior body to balance on the ball.

Starting Position
Lie face down on the stability ball with the ball under the stomach and hips (a). The hands are on the ground with the arms extended and the feet are on the ground. Press the hips slightly into the ball to stabilize the hips and spine and keep the abdominals engaged (as though to lift the abs inward and away from the ball).

Movement
Lift the left leg off the ground by squeezing the left glute and then lift the opposite arm (b). Hold for a moment and then repeat with the other arm and leg. The height of the lift isn't as important as maintaining stability. When starting this exercise, lift the leg first, then once stable, add the arm. When comfortable, lift both the arm and the leg at the same time.

Standing Exercises

The exercises presented here are standing exercises. These are considered completely unsupported because you are required to stabilize the body from the feet all the way up to the head. The only points of contact are your feet. I highly recommend starting these exercises with a wide stance because a wide base of support will feel most secure and stable. As you become more proficient and want a greater challenge you can begin to narrow your stance until your feet are together. As you are asked to do more, and eventually to add motion, you'll find your body being more dynamic. This is the final stage of the program. It's the culmination of everything you've been building toward. Keep your spine stable in every position and through every motion. These are the motions that will most closely simulate activities of daily life and leisure activities.

The first few exercises in this section require the use of an exercise tube or band. Sometimes these exercises are referred to as *de-rotation* or *anti-rotation* exercises because the resistance comes from only one side. Your body will need to resist the pull (torque and twist) by keeping your spine and core stable while performing the given exercise.

I prefer using tubes for these exercises because the handles make it easier to hold. Tubes that are wrapped with a protective sleeve are best because if they break, they won't snap back at you and cause injury. A few brands I trust are First Place Safety Toners or ProElite Covered Tubes. In terms of resistance level, start with a light tube and you can increase resistance as you progress. Be careful when you use tubes. When used properly, they will last a long time causing no issues.

Also, for these tube exercises, you will need to have the tube anchored to a wall or doorway. The tubing can be looped around an object such as a banister or another strong object that won't fall when force is applied to it. My recommendation is to get a door anchor. It is a device with a loop at one end that the tube can slip through and a plug or knot on the other that can be secured in a closed door. It is best to use a door that swings away from you. That way there is no chance that the door will open up as you pull the tube. Another recommendation is that you insert it on the hinge side of the doorway. That way the door would need to be opened at least 40 degrees before the door anchor would come loose.

Tube Press-Out

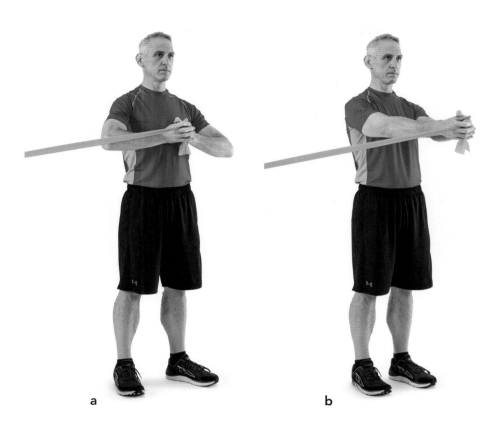

a   b

Objective
To activate the core and spinal stabilizers throughout the exercise.

Equipment
Tubing and door anchor

Starting Position
Stand sideways to the tube and at a distance so there is slight resistance on the tube. Hold the handle in the hands in front of the sternum or chest (a).

Movement
Engage the core and extend the arms out in front of the body (b). Hold this position for three to five seconds, then bring the hands back in to the chest. Repeat this exercise with the opposite side, making sure both the right and left sides have faced the anchor point. Make sure to keep the torso still during this exercise and do not let the tube twist the body toward the anchor.

Tube Circle

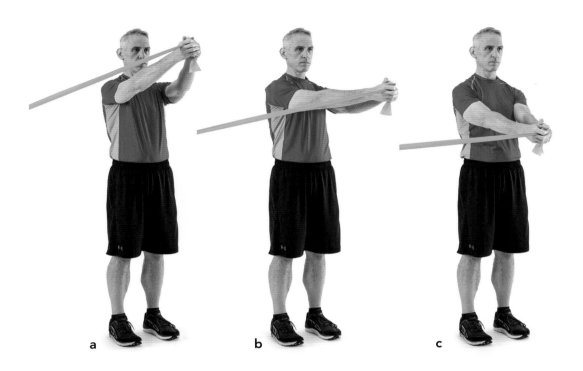

a   b   c

Objective
To activate the core and spinal stabilizers throughout the exercise.

Equipment
Tubing and door anchor

Starting Position
Stand sideways to the tube and at a distance, with slight resistance on the tube. With the handle in the hands, engage the core and extend the arms out in front of the body, keeping the hands right in front of the sternum or chest (a).

Movement
Hold the extended position and draw imaginary circles with the hands (b and c). You can also draw imaginary figure eights. Repeat this exercise with the opposite side, making sure both the right and left sides have faced the anchor point. Keep the torso still during this exercise and do not let the tube twist the body toward the anchor.

Tube Walk-Out

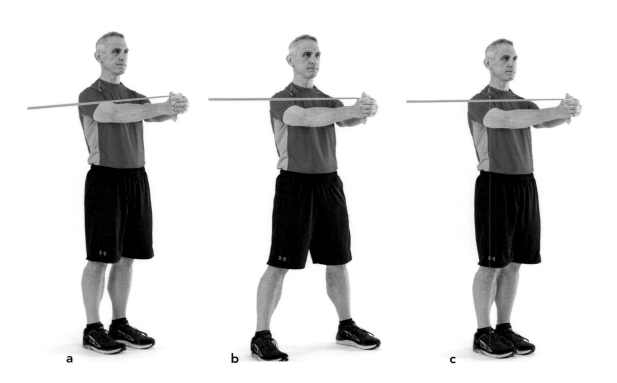

a   b   c

Objective
To activate the core and spinal stabilizers throughout the exercise.

Equipment
Tubing and door anchor

Starting Position
Stand sideways to the tube and at a distance, with slight resistance on the tube. Hold the handle in the hands in front of the sternum or chest (*a*).

Movement
With the handle in the hands, engage the core and extend the arms out in front of the body. Once the arms are extended and you are stable, take a step sideways away from the anchor point (*b*), hold for a moment, then step back toward the anchor point (*c*). Repeat this exercise with the opposite side, making sure both the right and left sides have faced the anchor point. If this feels too easy, take two steps away from the anchor point and return. The key is to keep the arms directly in front of the chest. Keep the torso still during this exercise and do not let the tube twist the body toward the anchor. Repeat this exercise with the opposite side, making sure both the right and left sides have faced the anchor point.

Tube Single-Arm Row

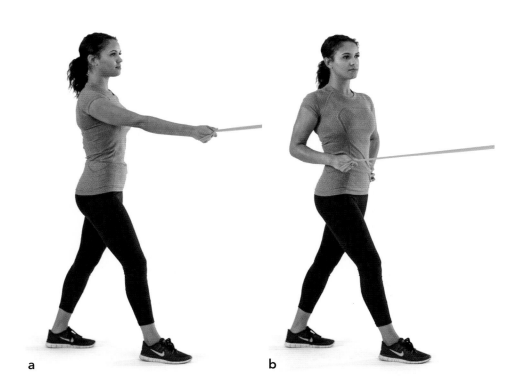

a   b

Objective
To activate the spinal erectors and stabilizers, as well as the posterior shoulder girdle (latissimus dorsi, trapezius, rhomboids, and posterior deltoids) throughout the exercise.

Equipment
Tubing and door anchor

Starting Position
Stand facing the anchor point in a straddle stance with one foot in front of the other, far enough apart to feel stable (a). Hold the handle in the hand that is on the same side as the forward foot.

Movement
Pull the handle toward the body keeping the elbow close (b), then return to the starting position. Continue for a specific number of repetitions before performing the exercise on the other side. Make sure to keep the hips and the torso still during this exercise and do not let the tube twist the body toward the anchor. It is all right if the shoulders turn slightly at the end of the movement as long as the core remains still. It is easy to make this a bigger motion than it needs to be.

Tube Single-Arm Press

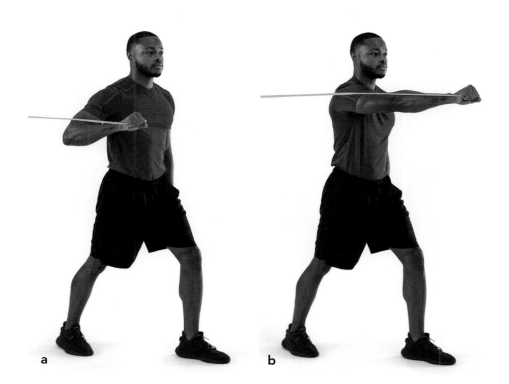

a   b

Objective
To activate the spinal stabilizers as well as the anterior shoulder girdle (pectoralis major, anterior deltoid, triceps, and serratus anterior).

Equipment
Tubing and door anchor

Starting Position
Face away from the anchor point and assume a staggered stance with one foot in front of the other, far enough apart to feel stable (a). Hold the handle in the hand opposite the forward foot and level with the chest, with the elbow out slightly away from the body. The shoulders should be parallel to the doorway and perpendicular (90 degrees) to the anchor point.

Movement
Fully press the handle away from the body, similar to a chest press (b), then return to the starting position. Make sure to keep the hips and torso still during this exercise and do not let the tube twist the body toward the anchor. Continue for a specific number of repetitions before performing the exercise on the other side.

Clock Step

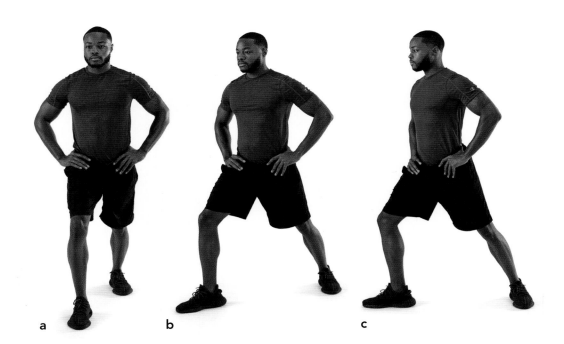

a   b   c

Objective
To move the body through space while keeping the core engaged and still. The rotation in this dynamic exercise will come from the hips, not from the waist.

Starting Position
Stand facing forward with the core slightly engaged and with the feet narrow and parallel to one another.

Movement
Take a step forward allowing the weight to transfer onto the forward foot (a), then return to the starting position. Consider this as 12 o'clock. Next, take a step with your foot aiming for two o'clock (b), allowing the weight to transfer onto the forward foot and return. Do the same for three o'clock (c). This is considered one repetition. Alternate with the opposite foot aiming for 12 o'clock, 10 o'clock, and nine o'clock.

Stand-Up–Sit-Down

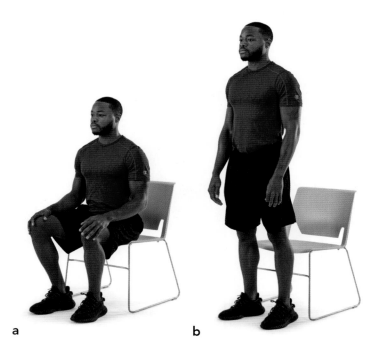

a   b

Objective
To challenge the core and spinal stabilizers and engage the lower extremities.

Equipment
Chair

Starting Position
Sit tall in a chair (or on the edge of a bed) with the feet flat on the floor and the knees bent so that the feet are under the body and the knees are right over the toes (a).

Movement
With the core stable and engaged, simply stand up (b), then sit back down again. Bend forward from the hips, and not the back, as much as possible without leaning over too far by rounding the back. Make sure to push down with the legs into the ground to stand, as this will activate the large leg muscles and transfer some of the responsibility from the low back to the legs. Over time, find places to sit in which the starting position is lower and lower until you are at a height that the knees and hips are at approximately 90 degrees with the ground.

Variation
Try it with one leg. With the core stable and engaged, stand up using both legs, then balance on one leg for a moment before slowly sitting back down using a single leg. Remember to keep most of your weight in your heel as you sit down to engage more of your hamstrings and glutes.

Step-Up

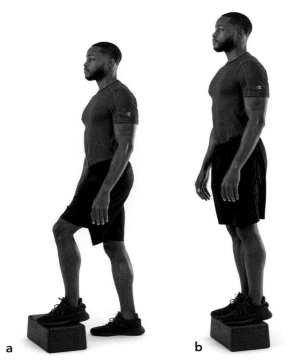

a   b

Objective
To activate the entire lower extremities while keeping the spine neutral and stable.

Equipment
A step or stairs in your home. The step should be approximately 8 inches high (average stair height).

Starting Position
Face the step and place one foot on the first step (*a*). Use the banister for balance if needed.

Movement
Step up onto the first step; balance at the top of the movement for a second by holding the opposite foot up and not placing it down on the step (*b*). Then step down to the starting position and repeat with the other foot. Make sure to establish balance on each repetition.

These exercises complete the partially supported, unsupported, and dynamic section of the exercises. Not all of these exercises may be included in your exercise prescription because every condition has its own set of exercises. In this chapter and the previous one, we focus primarily on spinal stabilization exercises in various positions. In the next chapter we look at exercises that focus on mobility and flexibility.

CHAPTER 6

Mobility and Flexibility Exercises

A small debate has been taking place in the fitness community over the past few years. Which is more important—stability or mobility? My stance and reasoning is this: Too much mobility and too little stability results in hyper-mobility. While this sounds fine, it can lead to injuries because the joints are forced into unnatural ranges of motion that weren't meant for our body's blueprint. However, on the other hand, too little mobility and too much stability can lead to rigidity, or joints that are supertight. This is seen in people who have very tight muscles and limited flexibility, which is also not ideal. These individuals will be overstabilized and won't move well, which creates poor body mechanics and leads to injury.

Much like Goldilocks and the Three Bears, each person's stability and mobility requirements need to be just right. We focus on the stability aspect first because without proper stability, the joints won't work properly. Then we begin to add exercises that fall into mobility training, which are the ones we discuss next. Remember, not every exercise is appropriate for every condition. Make sure to follow the guidelines based on *your* condition as outlined in part III.

Mobility Exercises

The exercises presented here focus on mobility, which is simply the ability to move. As discussed previously, every joint in the body has a natural range of motion based on its design, location, and adjacent parts. Certain joints will be limited by other bones in the area or muscles and ligaments that may be in the way.

If you watch a child move, you see such freedom of motion. Their bodies don't have years of compensatory faulty movement patterns. They move freely and take advantage of their natural range of motion. This mobility is often taken for granted until we lose it. When I was younger, I never stretched. I would work out and then shower and change without giving a single thought to stretching. Now, it's a different story. I spend a lot of my workout session trying to increase my mobility with full range of motion exercises and stretches.

Something to remember, however, is that mobility and stability are two sides of the same coin. While opposite in definition, they are both very important in achieving effortless and efficient movement. But which do you focus on first and why? Stability comes first in most situations. As previously discussed, if a joint or series of joints, like the spine, isn't stable, it can become hypermobile, meaning it has too great a range of motion and has difficulty being used in a safe controlled way. I have worked with many dancers who fall into this category. They have worked hard to maximize their range of motion, but once they are finished with their career and their bodies no longer need that range of motion, many of them experience dysfunction in their hips, knees, and SI joints. They need to work on stabilizing the joints so that they perform properly and so that there is sufficient tension within the joint at rest and in motion.

Picture a drawbridge. In order for a drawbridge to work properly, it first needs to be successful at being a bridge. It needs to have support to stay upright and withstand the forces of the wind and sea, not to mention the weight of the vehicles that cross it. It needs to be stable. In order to make the drawbridge work there needs to be just enough tension and strength from the pulleys to raise and lower the deck under the effect of gravity. If that deck is brought back too far and suddenly there is no tension on the deck against gravity, disaster awaits: At best, it won't be able to return to its original position, but at worst, it will tip over backward. Then you have a real problem. You put the surrounding joints into a compromised position when you have too great a range of motion in either your hips or spine. Also remember that going beyond your joints' natural range of motion will often damage the structure of the joints themselves. There is a reason we aren't meant to stretch beyond a certain point. So, stability needs to come first. Once a joint is stable, then we can begin to work on stretching and mobilizing it. Another factor to remember is that there are some joints that need a special focus on stability, such as the lumbar spine, while other joints will need added attention on mobility, such as the hip and thoracic spine.

The following mobility exercises will be added to your routine as you progress and may not be included in the first few weeks of training, which focus primarily on stability. Add in these mobility exercises as you become more stable in your spine.

Cat and Cow

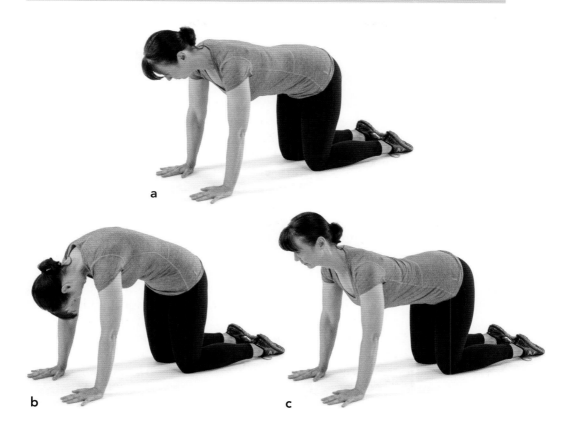

Objective
To work on the mobility and fluidity of the spine through flexion and extension.

Starting Position
Assume a quadruped position with a neutral spine (refer to Quadruped Hold on page 76 for a detailed description of this position) (a).

Movement
Initiate the cat portion of the move with a pelvic tilt (tucking the tailbone under) and rounding the back up to the sky (b). Move into the cow portion of the exercise by arching the back, bringing the chest toward the ground, and sticking the rear end in the air (c). A colleague of mine, Sue Hitzmann, calls this Sad Puppy, Happy Puppy: the sad puppy with the tail tucked under and the head down, and the happy puppy with the tail and the head up. Stay within a comfortable range of motion.

Side-Lying Telescope Arms

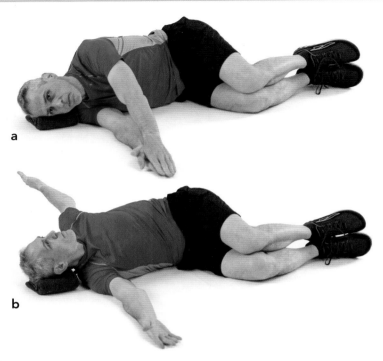

a

b

Objective
To promote thoracic rotation, allowing the midback to turn easier and take pressure off the lumbar spine.

Starting Position
This exercise can be performed two ways, depending on your condition and comfort level. For those who need to be in a posterior pelvic tilt and whose spine needs to be kept in a more flexed position, lie on the right side with both knees bent and hips at 90 degrees (a). For those who need to be in more of an anterior pelvic tilt and whose spine needs to be in an extension, lie on the right side with both legs straight, with the top foot about 12 inches in front of the bottom one. Use a pillow to support the head. Both arms should be out in front of the chest with the hands on top of one another.

Movement
Initiate the movement by taking the top arm and dragging it along the bottom arm, across the chest and then out to the side, creating a T with the arms and shoulders (b). The goal is to get the shoulder on the ground, or as close to the ground as possible, which will result in the rotation of the upper torso and shoulders while the hips remain still. Return to the starting position by bringing the arm in and dragging it along the chest and along the bottom arm again, this time reaching the top hand beyond the bottom hand. This should be done slowly and under control. Continue for a specific number of repetitions before performing the exercise on the other side.

Standing Telescope Arms

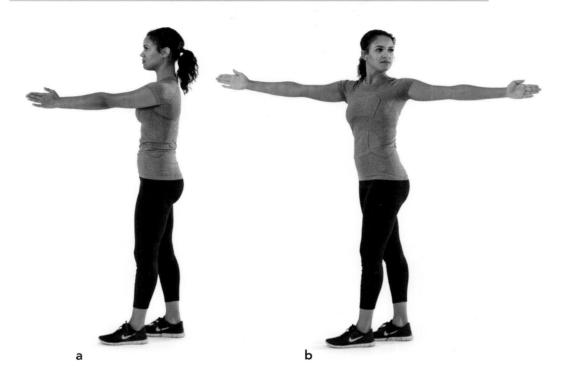

a   b

Objective
To promote thoracic rotation, allowing the midback to turn easier and take pressure off the lumbar spine.

Starting Position
Stand with the right side of the body against a wall. The arms are straight out in front of the chest and the hands are together. The left foot is slightly in front of the right foot (a).

Movement
Drag the left hand along the right arm, then the chest, and then out toward the wall behind, creating a T, while reaching forward with the right arm at the same time (b). The goal is to get the left shoulder on the wall, resulting in the rotation of the upper torso and the shoulders while the hips remain still. Return to the starting position by bringing the arm in and dragging it along the chest and along the right arm again, but this time reaching the left hand beyond the right hand. This should be done slowly and under control. Don't worry about the range of motion, it will come in time. Continue for a specific number of repetitions before performing the exercise on the other side.

Chicken Wing

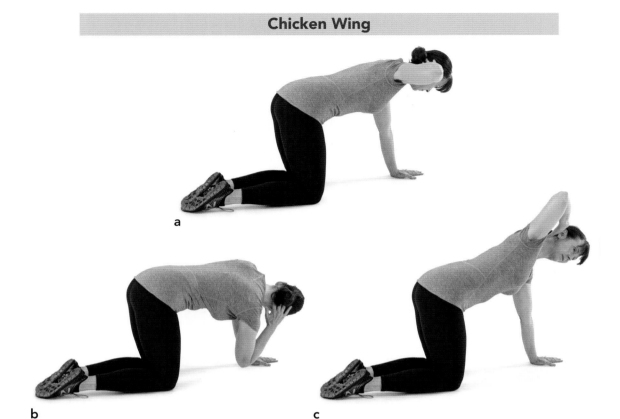

a

b   c

Objective
To promote thoracic rotation, allowing the midback to turn easier and take pressure off the lumbar spine.

Starting Position
Assume a quadruped position with a neutral spine (refer back to Quadruped Hold on page 76 for a detailed description of this position). Place one hand behind the head with the elbow out to the side (*a*).

Movement
Bring the elbow toward the ground and slightly back, aiming for the elbow to go through the space made by the opposite arm and thigh, as if threading a needle (*b*). Switch directions by rotating the upper spine bringing that elbow up toward the sky, turning the chest outward at the same time (*c*). Don't worry if the range of motion isn't very great. Continue for a specific number of repetitions before performing the exercise on the other side.

Tail Wag

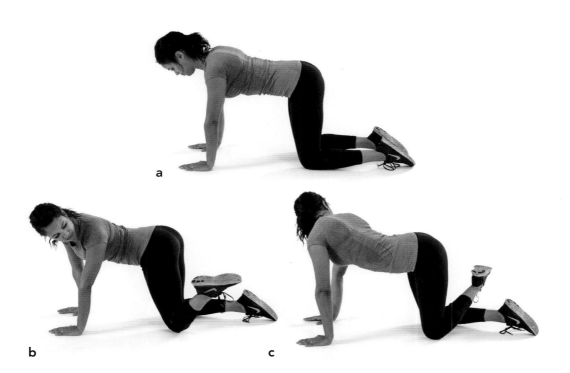

a

b   c

Objective
To promote greater lateral flexibility in the spine.

Starting Position
Assume a quadruped position with a neutral spine (refer back to Quadruped Hold on page 76 for a detailed description of this position) (*a*). Lift the left foot off the ground while keeping the left knee on the ground.

Movement
Rotate the lifted leg so the left foot moves away from the opposite leg. At the same time, turn the head and look at the lifted foot; the spine should side bend (laterally flex) to the left (*b*). Then do the opposite, bringing the left foot across the opposite leg and looking over to the right while side bending to the right (*c*). The side-to-side movement should feel like a tail wagging. Continue for a specific number of repetitions before alternating sides.

Articulating Bridge

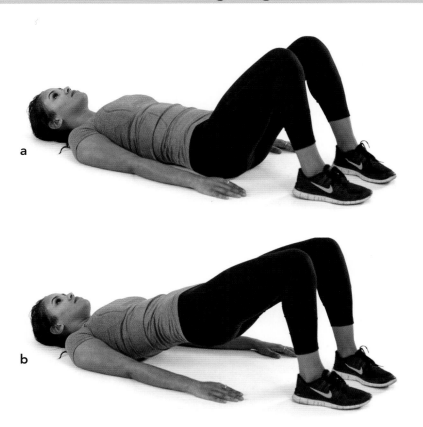

a

b

Objective
To promote spinal flexion and articulation.

Starting Position
Lie on the back with the knees bent at 90 degrees and the feet flat on the floor
(*a*).

Movement
Using the abdominals, move the pelvis into a posterior tilt and slowly peel the
hips and spine off the floor one vertebra at a time (*b*). Don't arch the back or
lift the rib cage. In fact, keep the ribs on the ground for the first week or two
of training. It is common to lift too high and end up arching the back, causing
undue compression in the lumbar spine. Return to the starting position by trying
to put the spine back down one vertebra at a time, focusing on flexing the spine
on the way down and maintaining a pelvic tilt the entire time. Imagine lifting and
then placing a string of pearls down on a table, one pearl at a time.

Sphinx

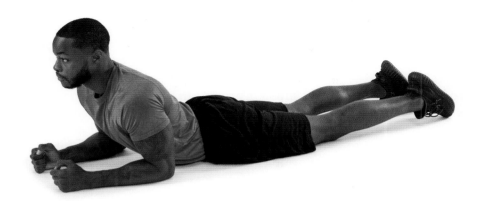

Objective
To promote thoracic extension. This is a very basic exercise that I often have my clients perform between sets of other exercises as a rest position. They have no idea that it is actually an important exercise for their upper back.

Starting Position
Lie on the stomach.

Movement
Prop up onto the elbows while keeping the hips on the ground. Relax through the shoulders; the shoulder blades may even come toward each other as they relax. Look forward and slightly upward. Hold the position for 30 seconds and repeat.

Stretching and Flexibility Exercises

The exercises presented here focus on stretching and flexibility. This is probably the most overlooked part of the equation. There are many reasons for this. These exercises can be uncomfortable and people want to avoid what doesn't feel good. Also, stretching comes at the end, and after people have finished exercises, they usually just want to get on with their day. And let's be honest: Some people just don't like to stretch! But it is a vital component to the process. Tight hip flexors and hamstrings can have a major impact on your lumbar spine, so stretching these areas needs to be given the same attention as the exercises meant to strengthen them. You should feel these stretches, but they should not be too uncomfortable. Your muscles should feel the pull and perhaps feel mildly uncomfortable, but it should be tolerable. On a scale of 1 to 10, with 10 being extreme pain, don't take the stretch beyond a 5 or a 6.

Kneeling Hip Flexor Stretch

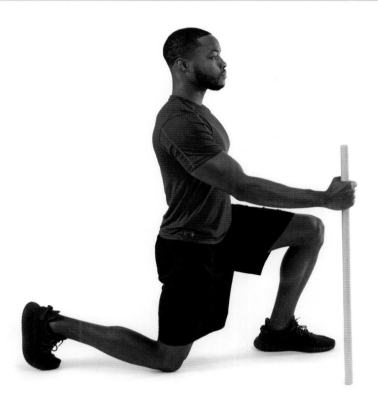

Objective
To stretch the front of the hip (hip flexors).

Starting Position
Assume a position with one knee on the ground and the opposite foot forward with both knees bent at approximately 90 degrees. Hold onto a chair or stick for balance if needed.

Movement
Tuck the tailbone and slowly draw the hips forward as if someone is pulling from the front pocket until a stretch is felt in the front of the leg. The range of motion won't be very great. Do not lunge too deep and exceed the point of stretch. Hold the stretch for 60 to 90 seconds, alternate sides, and repeat on the opposite side.

Doorway Hamstring Stretch

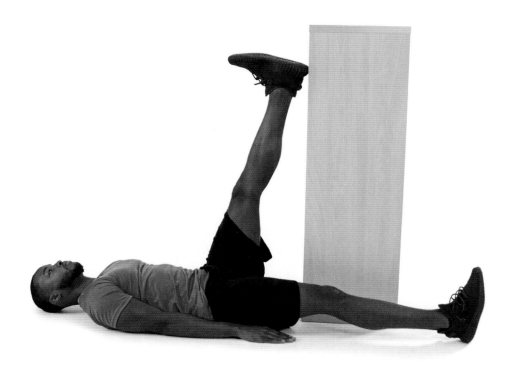

Objective
To stretch the backs of the legs (hamstrings).

Starting Position
Lie in a doorframe and place one leg up against the door jamb.

Movement
Keep the leg straight so that the stretch is felt in the back of the leg, preferably in the hamstrings, although some may feel it more strongly in the calf muscles. If there isn't much pull, get further into the doorway. If it is too intense or you can't straighten out the leg, back up a little. Try to relax into the stretch. Hold this stretch for 60 to 90 seconds, alternate sides, and repeat using the other leg.

Strap Hamstring Stretch

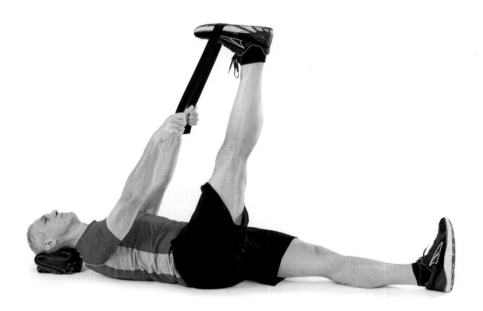

Objective
To stretch the backs of the legs (hamstrings).

Equipment
Strap, rope, or belt.

Starting Position
Lie on the back with a strap under the foot, holding the ends of the strap in each hand.

Movement
Lift the leg up by pulling the strap with the hands until a stretch is felt in the hamstrings. Keep the knee straight for this stretch; it is much more effective this way. At the beginning, the leg that stays on the ground can remain bent. As you progress, straighten it out to increase the intensity of the stretch. Hold for 60 to 90 seconds, alternate sides, and repeat.

Lying Lumbar Stretch

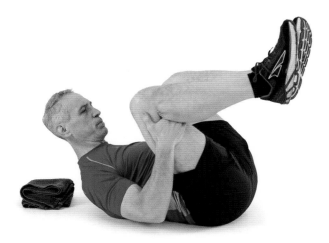

Objective
To stretch the low back.

Starting Position
Lie on the back.

Movement
Hug the knees into the chest and hold. For an advanced technique or for those with spondylolisthesis, perform this stretch with the Togu ball under the sacrum. Hold for 30 to 60 seconds and repeat.

Seated Lumbar Stretch

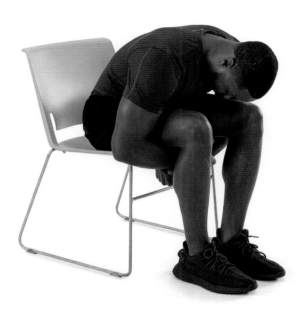

Objective
To stretch the low back.

Starting Position
Sit in a chair.

Movement
Fold the upper body forward over the thighs and hug the legs into the chest. Hold for 30 to 60 seconds and repeat.

Knee-to-Chest Stretch

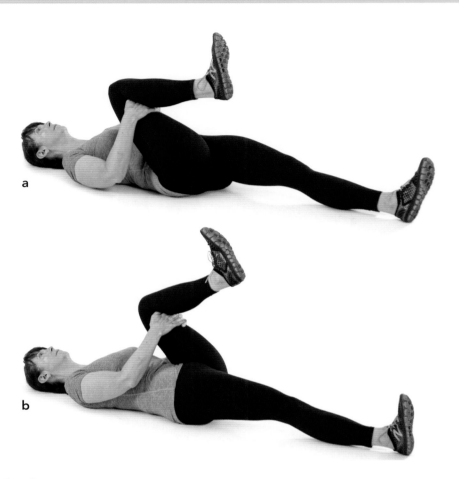

Objective
To stretch the upper hamstrings and low back.

Starting Position
Lie on the back with the knees bent at 90 degrees and with the feet flat on the floor.

Movement
Bring one knee into the chest and hug it by wrapping the hands or the arms around the thigh and hold (a). Hold for 30 to 60 seconds then repeat on the other side (b), alternating sides each time.

Adductor Stretch

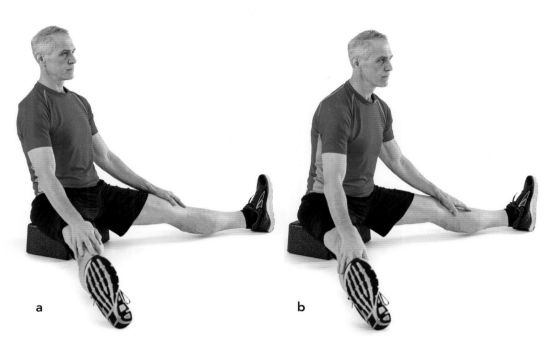

a   b

Objective
To stretch the inner thighs (adductor group). Believe it or not, the inner thighs are often tight and can affect the lower back.

Starting Position
Sit on the ground in a straddle position, legs in a wide V. Sitting on a step or a small stool may make this stretch easier and more comfortable (*a*). Spread the legs as wide as possible.

Movement
Sit up straight and lean forward while keeping the chest high (*b*). Try not to round the back while leaning forward. It is more important to sit up straight than to lean far forward. Hold this stretch for 60 to 90 seconds and repeat.

Supine Piriformis Stretch

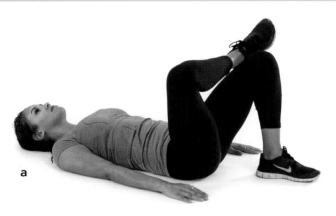

a

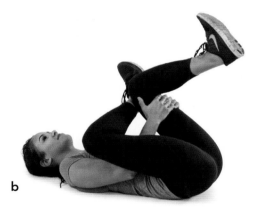

b

Objective
To stretch the piriformis and buttocks.

Starting Position
Lie on your back with the right ankle crossed over the left knee with the shin as perpendicular to the body as possible (a).

Movement
Hold onto the back of the left thigh with both hands and pull the leg toward the body until a stretch is felt (b). Hold for 30 to 60 seconds, alternate sides, and repeat with the legs switched.

Seated Piriformis Stretch

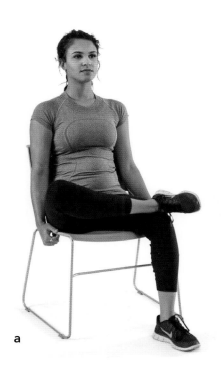

a

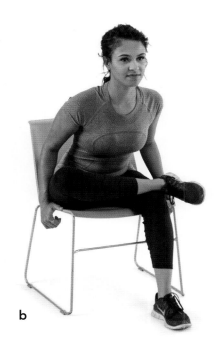

b

Objective
To stretch the piriformis and buttocks.

Starting Position
Sit in a chair with the right ankle crossed over the left knee with the shin as parallel to the floor as possible (a).

Movement
Sit up nice and tall and hold. Lean forward over the leg if more of a stretch is needed (b). Hold for 30 to 60 seconds and alternate sides to repeat.

Chest Stretch

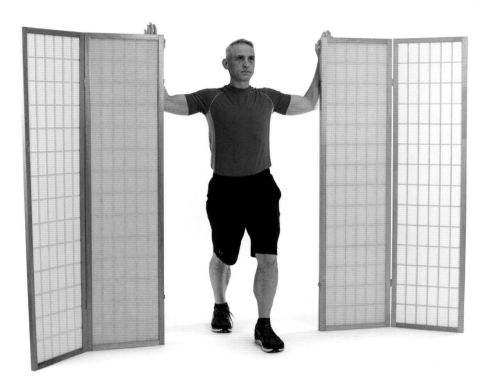

Objective
To stretch the anterior shoulder girdle (chest).

Starting Position
Stand inside a doorframe with the arms in a goalpost position, elbows bent at 90 degrees, and the forearms on the door frame.

Movement
Step through the doorway until you feel a stretch in the chest and hold. If this bothers the low back, don't step as far into the doorway; chances are, you went too far and are arching the back. Hold for 30 seconds and repeat.

I have said it before but it bears repeating: Not every exercise is meant for every body. Based on your specific lumbar condition, certain exercises are exactly what you need, while others will be contraindicated. The following chapters will discuss some of the most common spinal conditions and offer specific recommendations, from proper exercises and volume of exercise to when you should change the exercises as you become stronger.

PART III

Common Conditions

I can't tell you how often I hear "I have a bad back," or "I have low back pain," from a new client. These may be the most frequently heard phrases in my assessment process. The problem is, it doesn't tell me anything. It is too generic. If you went to a mechanic, would you say, "My car is broken"? Well . . . which part? What exactly is wrong? It's the same thing with your body. Simply saying your low back hurts doesn't convey enough information for me to help.

There is a myriad of conditions that could be involved when it comes to low back pain, from disc issues to spondylolisthesis to stenosis and beyond, and believe it or not, each one needs to be managed differently in regard to exercise. Remember the client I mentioned in chapter 3 who came in with the incomplete diagnosis of stenosis and anterolisthesis? For three weeks, she worked hard to manage her pain based on the information she had given me, but her pain kept growing. Then she brought in her MRI. We had been training her incorrectly based on her reported diagnosis of stenosis, but not on her spinal condition of spondylolisthesis. Once we had the correct diagnosis, she could do the correct exercises and was out of pain quickly and on the road to recovery, but all of that time was lost and she suffered unnecessarily. This example demonstrates why it's important to talk to your physician and make sure you have the proper diagnosis before jumping into an exercise program, so that you can do the right exercises for your specific condition.

The following chapters are organized by specific condition, starting first with nonspecific low back pain. We will define each condition, describe what has happened to the physical structures, discuss the contraindications to said condition, and then explain what you should do and which exercises will be appropriate for your condition. This will give you the road map needed to stabilize and strengthen your low back, and hopefully improve your quality of life. For additional information and selected videos explaining some of the foundational and more difficult exercises, you can visit www.backexercisebook.com.

This part of the book will be more detailed and scientific than previous chapters but don't be intimidated. It is very important that you understand the ins and outs of your condition, because only then will you be able to take control of it. The majority of clients don't understand very much about their condition or what it means. They may hear the terminology, but the condition either wasn't fully explained to them or it was explained in a language they didn't understand, and some are too embarrassed to ask further questions. It's your body. Understanding it is the key to healing it.

Straight Talk

Have you ever noticed that many professionals seem to speak in a language all their own? Professional jargon is common in every vocation, especially medicine. Some doctors tend to forget that we all didn't graduate from medical school. Even in my profession of exercise physiology and kinesiology, some personal trainers use big words, perhaps to impress clients or to generate confidence in their knowledge base, but I find it often leads to confusion rather than clarity. In these situations, I remind people that they need to be their own best advocate and ask for detailed explanations until they are fully satisfied that they understand the answer. Remember, the doctor works for you. You are paying for their time; get the most out of it.

Once you have a diagnosis of your condition, you need to understand what it is and explore the possible treatment options, whether they include surgery, epidural shots, therapy, or exercise. Every physician will have a preferred method of treatment and some of them are surgery-happy, so I always suggest getting a second opinion before jumping into surgery too quickly. I realize there is a temptation to move boldly to just get it done, often because the promise of quick pain relief is too enticing. But keep in mind that surgery will forever alter your structure. Things will never be as they were before you went under the knife. Back surgery is not something to take lightly; it can be a major surgery, so it is almost always worth at least considering or trying nonsurgical options first. Once you are comfortable with the treatment options you and your physician have determined, then you can move forward with it. For many, this book and the following chapters will be used to follow these treatment options.

The following chapters should serve as an explanation and a road map of what you can do now to help manage your low back pain. If you have completed some form of physical therapy, I hope that some of these exercises feel familiar to you. It is important that to read the entire chapter and not just jump into the exercises. Each chapter will educate you not only about your condition, but also about why you are doing the exercises that are listed. When you understand why you are doing a particular exercise or series of exercises, then you're more likely to be mindful and compliant while doing the exercises, and will therefore see greater results.

CHAPTER 7

Nonspecific Low Back Pain

More than 80 percent of people will experience low back pain at some point in their lifetime. That is an overwhelming majority of people. Low back pain (LBP) is the second most common reason for visiting a physician, right behind the common cold. If you are reading this, chances are you are currently suffering from low back pain or have suffered in the past. Optimally, you've already been given a diagnosis from the doctor and can skip to the chapter that applies to your condition. However, there are a large number of people with low back pain who don't have a specific condition or diagnosis. Their condition falls into the category of *generalized low back pain* or, more accurately, *nonspecific low back pain*.

Definition

Nonspecific low back pain is defined as low back pain that is not attributable to a recognizable, known specific pathology (e.g., infection, tumor, osteoporosis, lumbar spine fracture, structural deformity, inflammatory disorder, radicular syndrome, or cauda equina syndrome).[1] In other words, there's no specific source; it could be caused by many different factors.

Despite being so common, the number of people who don't go to the doctor when they suffer from LBP outnumber those who do go to the doctor by two to one.[2] LBP is not limited to any specific age or demographic. Men and women, young and old suffer equally from LBP. In fact, we are seeing an increase in the number of teenagers with low back pain.[3]

Causes

Many contributing factors can lead to low back pain. First, there are mechanical factors. Poor posture, faulty lifting technique, awkward movements such as twisting or bending, and repetitive motions like raking or shoveling can all lead to muscle strains or overuse injuries. These are rarely traumatic events, but are considered accumulation injuries. They are incidents that have taken place over a long period of time, but, much like the proverbial straw that broke the camel's back, the moment when your back has finally had enough is what is memorable.

Think of it like a house of cards. For years you have been setting up one card at a time. Each one is perfectly balanced, but standing precariously, until one day there's a sudden disturbance and the whole tower comes crashing down. Your back has been weakened over time and it takes only one event for it to give out. That single event didn't cause the back injury—it just tipped it over the edge.

Another factor that can lead to low back pain is being overweight or obese.[4] There are multiple reasons for this. First, increased weight applies more disc pressure. In addition, overweight or obese individuals tend to have stomachs that protrude farther out from the spinal column, increasing the pull on the lumbar spine toward lordosis (arching), and increasing pressure on the discs and the lumbar muscles (erectors, quadratus lumborum, spinal stabilizers) to keep the torso erect. We often see a weakness in an individual's core muscu-lature (think of all the muscles from the ribs to the buttocks) when someone suffers from low back pain. In this case it may be a question of whether the chicken or the egg came first. Did the weakness of the core muscles lead to low back pain or did the low back pain result in the muscles becoming weaker? The jury is still out on that. Either way, these are the muscles that you will be focusing on during your exercises.

There are lesser known factors that are also shown to have some correla-tion to low back pain. Smoking has been linked to low back pain, although the "how" remains a mystery.[5] Genetic and hereditary factors have also seen some relationship with low back pain, possibly due to arthritic factors passed down generationally. We also see low back pain among both those who do too little and those who do too much physical activity. Those who don't do any exercise and live a very sedentary lifestyle are as likely to develop low back pain as those who pursue highly strenuous physical activities, often without enough rest and recuperation before the next workout.[6]

Symptoms

Let's talk about severity and duration of pain. There are three categories when it comes to injury: acute (less than 6 weeks), subacute (6 to 12 weeks), and chronic (more than 12 weeks).[7] In only about 10 to 15 percent of acute cases does the low back pain become chronic.[8] With medication and time, the matter begins to resolve by itself, often waiting to rear its ugly head another day (remember the house of cards?). It is through proper exercise and strengthening that you can keep low back pain from recurring.

Without carefully orchestrated healing and strengthening, it is usually only a matter of time before low back pain returns; the frequency and duration of these episodes vary. However, strengthening the muscles and stabilizers may shorten the duration of pain episodes and space them farther and farther apart. Instead of experiencing debilitating pain for four to six weeks every few months, it can be reduced to 5 to 10 days every 9 to 12 months. Sometimes the back pain is held at bay for years, to the point that the client forgets about being injured at all.

Treatment Options

Physicians often treat low back pain with medication first: anti-inflammatories (NSAIDS), and, if needed, muscle relaxants. They may also suggest physical therapy, and if they do, I highly recommend it. A physical therapist will teach many of the exercises that you see in this book, and you will get hands-on learning and training that is tailored to your specific issues. I also recommend getting a large, good-quality gel ice pack, and particularly recommend the Chattanooga Colpac Oversized Ice Pack. I use the 12 inch by 18.5 inch size, but they have a variety of sizes. I have two in my freezer that I can rotate between, using a pack for 20 minutes at a time followed by 40 minutes off, and then repeating.

Other suggested treatment methods include chiropractic, acupuncture, and manual therapy (massage). All of these have some benefit depending on the issue, patient, and practitioner. There is no one-size-fits-all cure. Although the science is divided when it comes to nontraditional forms of therapy, there is a lot of anecdotal evidence that supports it. I agree with that point of view. I've known many people who have had success working with massage therapists, chiropractors, and acupuncturists, and would recommend these therapies as long as it is discussed with your doctor and a responsible practitioner is chosen.

Straight Talk

"I have no time to ice my back," say many clients. But there are always moments to ice. I use my morning and afternoon commute to ice my back or other needy body regions. Remember that icing provides benefits beyond the time when the ice is on the body. Icing can promote long-term reduction of inflammation when done regularly. In the morning, I put an ice pack behind my back during my 30- to 40-minute commute. The first few minutes are tough, but I get used to it quickly and then forget it is even there. Once at work, I am lucky to have a freezer so I put the pack in there and repeat on my way home. This way, I don't forget, and it is done multiple times daily. If I try to remember to ice at the end of the day at home, I often forget. This method has become a habit and part of my normal routine. Whether you have been sedentary all day, or lifting, twisting, and bending, remember that both types of activities can equally cause inflammation in your low back. Icing is one of the easiest ways to reduce the inflammation. Make sure you plan the time to do it.

Training Focus

The exercise programs described in tables 7.1 through 7.6 will work best for those who are not in an acute state of low back pain. If you are experiencing spasms or having extreme low back pain, wait until the symptoms have subsided a bit before starting. If you have already seen a physician or physical therapist, and need a strengthening or maintenance program that will help to prevent future episodes, then these exercises are for you. Again, I don't recommend that you begin these exercises while you're experiencing back spasms. The exercises will be counterproductive; you need to be patient and wait until things have relaxed a bit. Then the exercises will have much greater benefit. Each month, you will either add new exercises or replace some of your current exercises with more advanced ones. The goal is progression. You want to make progress, and the only way to do that is to work a little harder by adjusting one of the variables. Those variables are volume (the number of sets and repetitions, or total number of exercises), load (the amount of weight being lifted), and frequency (the number of exercise days per week). Each month, you can look forward to a change in your exercise program, and as long as you are not experiencing any increased pain, you will keep up with the new exercise program until the next month. If you have increased pain, go back to the previous month for another week, then give the new exercise program another try.

Keep in mind that not all exercises are meant for everybody. There may be an exercise that works well for one person but may cause another person significant discomfort. Simply stop and avoid the exercise that hurts. Return to that exercise later in the month or even the following month to see if you have become strong enough to do it without pain. From my personal and professional experience, there may be an exercise that you will never be able to do, and that's okay. If you cannot perform this one exercise, it will not make or break your success. Do the ones that don't cause you pain.

Let's discuss what kind of pain is okay and what kind is not. Normally, we instruct our clients that a little discomfort is acceptable. On a scale of 1 to 10, with 1 being no pain at all and a 10 being the worst pain you can imagine, where would you rank your pain as you perform an exercise? If it is a 1 to a 3, it is okay to work through it. This would include some mild discomfort. However, if the pain is severe, don't perform the exercise that day. You may feel some pain with the first or second repetition of an exercise and want to immediately stop. I encourage you to do a couple more repetitions and see if the pain dissipates. It often will. However, if the pain continues above level 3, don't push through. Let it go for the day, and move on to the next exercise.

You will begin by getting comfortable with the exercises and establishing the habit of doing them regularly. I often tell my clients that I want them to do the exercises every day. It sounds like a lot but let's face reality: Most people will do the exercises three to four times per week. That's perfect. However, when I tell them to do it three to four times per week, they may do it only once or twice. Success hinges on your consistency. The more you do it, the stronger you will get.

Before You Begin: Finding Neutral Spine and Engaging Kegels

Neutral spine was first discussed in detail back in chapter 1, but it is worth repeating because it applies specifically to your nonspecific low back pain and the exercises prescribed in the following program. When talking about low back pain, neutral spine is the spinal position you can maintain with little to no pain. The following exercises should be performed in a pain-free neutral spine.

The clinical definition of *neutral spine* is the position in which the anterior superior iliac spine is on the same plane as the posterior superior iliac spine. While those anatomical landmarks mean something to many health care professionals, they don't translate nearly as well to the general population. For the rest of us, neutral spine is the position in which your spine has the least amount of stress on it, where the curves of the cervical, thoracic, and lumbar regions support each other and are able to cushion the spine optimally. We will focus primarily on the lumbar spine, but remember that if you change the angle of one region, the others will also change, for better or worse.

Try to think of traditional neutral spine as having not too high of an arch in the back and not too little. If you are lying on the ground, place your hand under the low back. Is there a lot of space? If it represents the Golden Gate Bridge rather than a footbridge over a small koi pond, then it's too big. You need to bring your ribs down a bit toward your hips and flatten out your back a little. If this is uncomfortable for your head and neck, and results in a large arch in your neck, put a pillow or rolled up towel under your neck to keep it as neutral as possible as well. Alternately, if your back is completely flattened to the floor, this isn't ideal either. There should be a little bit of an arch, high enough so that your fingers can get under your back but not your whole hand, and definitely not your whole fist. If this traditional neutral spine is uncomfortable or causes pain, modify the position so that it feels comfortable. As you become stronger, try to get closer to the traditional neutral spine position.

You will see that your first exercise in month 1 is to find your neutral spine and maintain it. Lie down (supine) on your back in a position that produces little to no pain, or such that the pain subsides as you continue relaxing on your back. Next, find your Kegel muscles. These are usually described as the muscles that help to hold back a stream of urine. They are your pelvic floor muscles, a muscle group that comprises part of your inner core, and they should be slightly engaged during these exercises. Don't grip them hard, just a light hold: think 30 percent of your maximum. Hold for about 20 to 30 seconds. As you become stronger, it will become easier to maintain. Focus on keeping the pelvic floor muscles engaged throughout each exercise. It may not be easy, and you may forget. Once you can find neutral spine and engage the pelvic floor muscles, it's time to move on to the exercises.

Table 7.1   Month 1 Exercises

1. Neutral spine and Kegel		Hold for 30 sec	
2. Bent-knee fallout		2 sets of 10 reps each side	Page 55
3. Heel slide		2 sets of 10 reps each side	Page 56
4. Marching		2 sets of 10 reps each side (alternating)	Page 57
5. Lying overhead reach (single- or double-arm)		2 sets of 15 reps on each side. For low back pain, do either the single- or double-arm version as long as you maintain good posture and don't arch the back.	Page 63
6. Pelvic press hold		5 sec hold for 5 reps	Page 70
7. Pelvic press hip extension		2 sets of 10 reps each side (alternating)	Page 71
8. Pelvic press shoulder retraction		5 reps of 5 sec hold for 2 sets	Page 72

Table 7.1   Month 1 Exercises

9. Togu pelvic tilt		2 sets of 12 reps	Page 65
10. Kneeling hip flexor stretch		30 sec hold for 2 reps each side	Page 111
11. Doorway hamstring stretch or strap hamstring stretch		60 sec hold for 2 reps each side	Page 112 or 113
12. Knee-to-chest stretch		30 sec hold for 2 reps each side	Page 116
13. Seated side bend		2 sec hold for 12 reps each side	Page 86

Table 7.2   Month 2 Exercises

1. March-up		2 sets of 8 reps each side (alternating)	Page 58
2. Leg lowering		2 sets of 10 reps each side (alternating)	Page 59
3. Dying bug		2 sets of 8 reps each side	Page 61
4. Clamshell		2 sets of 15 reps each side	Page 62
5. Pelvic press hip extension (with opposite-arm lift when you feel ready)		2 sets of 8 reps each side (alternating)	Page 71
6. Pelvic press shoulder retraction		8 reps of 5 sec hold for 2 sets	Page 72
7. Pelvic press W		5 reps of 5 sec hold for 2 sets	Page 73
8. Articulating bridge		2 sets of 10 reps	Page 108
9. Kneeling hip flexor stretch		30 sec hold for 2 reps each side	Page 111

Table 7.2 Month 2 Exercises

10. Strap hamstring stretch		30 sec hold for 2 reps each side	Page 113
11. Knee-to-chest stretch		30 sec hold for 2 reps each side	Page 116
12. Supine or seated piriformis stretch		30 sec hold for 2 reps each side	Page 118 or 119

Table 7.3 Month 3 Exercises

1. Leg lowering		2 sets of 15 reps each side (alternating)	Page 59
2. Dying bug		2 sets of 15 reps each side	Page 61
3. Advanced kick-out		2 sets of 10 reps each side	Page 60

(Continued)

Table 7.3   **Month 3 Exercises** *(continued)*

4. Full plank		3 reps of 10 sec hold for 2 sets with 3 sec rest between reps	Page 82
5. Side plank (on knees if needed)		15 sec hold for 2 reps each side	Page 83
6. Quadruped hold with opposite-arm tap		2 sets of 12 reps each side	Page 77
7. Quadruped hip extension lift		2 sets of 12 reps each side	Page 79
8. Tail wag		2 sets of 15 reps each side	Page 107
9. Standing telescope arms		2 sets of 8 reps each side	Page 105
10. Kneeling hip flexor stretch		30 sec hold for 2 reps each side	Page 111

Table 7.3   Month 3 Exercises

11. Strap hamstring stretch		30 sec hold for 2 reps each side	Page 113
12. Knee-to-chest stretch		30 sec hold for 2 reps each side	Page 116
13. Supine or seated piriformis stretch		30 sec hold for 2 reps each side	Page 118 or 119

Table 7.4   Month 4 Exercises

1. Dying bug		2 sets of 15 reps each side	Page 61
2. Advanced kick-out		2 sets of 10 reps each side	Page 60
3. Full plank		3 reps of 10 sec hold for 2 sets with 3 sec rest between reps	Page 82
4. Side plank		20 sec hold for 2 reps each side	Page 83

(Continued)

Table 7.4   Month 4 Exercises *(continued)*

5. Stability ball seated hip shift		2 sets of 15 reps each side	Page 87
6. Stability ball seated knee lift		2 sets of 10 reps each side	Page 88
7. Stability ball hip extension hold		6 reps of 5 sec hold for 2 sets each side. Focus on a small range of motion, and do not arch the back.	Page 90
8. Quadruped birddog		2 sets of 8 reps each side	Page 80
9. Stand-up–sit-down		2 sets of 20 reps	Page 99
10. Standing telescope arms		2 sets of 8 reps each side	Page 105

Table 7.4   Month 4 Exercises

11. Kneeling hip flexor stretch		30 sec hold for 2 reps each side	Page 111
12. Strap hamstring stretch		30 sec hold for 2 reps each side	Page 113
13. Knee-to-chest stretch		30 sec hold for 2 reps each side	Page 116
14. Supine or seated piriformis stretch		30 sec hold for 2 reps each side	Page 118 or 119

Table 7.5   Month 5 Exercises

1. Full plank		30 sec hold for 3 reps	Page 82
2. Side plank		30 sec hold for 3 reps each side	Page 83

(Continued)

Table 7.5   Month 5 Exercises *(continued)*

3. Articulating bridge		2 sets of 15 reps	Page 108
4. Tube press-out		2 sets of 15 reps each side	Page 93
5. Tube circle		2 sets of 15 reps each side in both directions	Page 94
6. Tube walk-out		2 sets of 15 reps each side	Page 95
7. Clock step		2 sets of 5 reps each direction (12, 2, & 3 o'clock; then 12, 10, & 9 o'clock)	Page 98
8. Stability ball seated knee lift		2 sets of 12 reps each side	Page 88

Table 7.5   Month 5 Exercises

9. Chicken wing		2 sets of 10 reps each side	Page 106
10. Kneeling hip flexor stretch		30 sec hold for 2 reps each side	Page 111
11. Strap hamstring stretch		30 sec hold for 2 reps each side	Page 113
12. Knee-to-chest stretch		30 sec hold for 2 reps each side	Page 116
13. Supine or seated piriformis stretch		30 sec hold for 2 reps each side	Page 118 or 119
14. Adductor stretch		30 sec hold for 2 reps	Page 117

Table 7.6   Month 6 Exercises

1. Full plank		45 sec hold for 3 reps	Page 82
2. Side plank		30 sec hold for 3 reps each side	Page 83
3. Articulating bridge		2 sets of 15 reps	Page 108
4. Tube circle		2 sets of 15 reps each side in both directions	Page 94
5. Tube walk-out		2 sets of 15 reps each side	Page 95
6. Stand-up–sit-down (single-leg)		2 sets of 8 reps. For low back pain, if single leg is too difficult, perform using both legs.	Page 99

Table 7.6   Month 6 Exercises

7. Side-lying telescope arms		2 sets of 12 reps each side	Page 104
8. Sphinx		30 sec hold for 2 reps	Page 109
9. Chicken wing		2 sets of 10 reps each side	Page 106
10. Stability ball seated knee lift		2 sets of 12 reps each side	Page 88
11. Stability ball walk-out		2 sets of 12 reps. Begin walk-out with posterior tilt.	Page 89

(Continued)

Table 7.6 Month 6 Exercises *(continued)*

12. Kneeling hip flexor stretch		30 sec hold for 2 reps each side	Page 111
13. Strap hamstring stretch		30 sec hold for 2 reps each side	Page 113
14. Supine or seated piriformis stretch		30 sec hold for 2 reps each side	Page 118 or 119
15. Adductor stretch		30 sec hold for 2 reps	Page 117
16. Chest stretch		30 sec hold for 2 reps	Page 120

Continuing Your Training

By the end of the sixth month, you should be able to manage your low back pain with the exercises given. Be mindful of remaining stable in your core throughout any exercise activity. I highly recommend the use of machines in this phase of training because they are a relatively safe way to get back into lifting weights. They put you in a dedicated path of motion, which eliminates some of the inherent instability of free weights. This may go against what some trainers have told you in the past, but you are now reintroducing your body to weight training and if you ask your body to stabilize too many things at one time (e.g., your core and spine, hips, legs, knees, scapula, arms), your body may not be ready and it may fail and send you backward. Keep in mind that this is temporary, and you can and should reintroduce free weights to your routine as you get stronger in the weeks and months to come. This will challenge you to stabilize in many different planes of motion and will be an important part of strength building once you're ready. Also, don't forget to train your lower body—your hips and legs support the low back more than you realize. Exercises such as the weighted step-up, squat, and lunge are perfect for someone who has nonspecific low back pain because you don't have the same limitations as those with other spinal conditions.

Also, you should now be able to do group exercise classes such as Pilates, yoga, or stretching, but be cautious. While class instructors have the best of intentions, they may ask you to do more than what your spine is capable of at this time. Start slow and listen to your body. If a little voice inside is telling you to stop, listen to it. You don't want your pain to flare up again.

I realize, too, that not everyone belongs to a gym. In that case, you can continue to do months 5 and 6 exercises indefinitely if you choose. But remember that the body gets used to what it does regularly and will stagnate and weaken over time if you don't change things up a bit. You can always increase reps, sets, or even hold times to jazz it up a bit. To challenge your body, I suggest one of the following two options for month 7 and beyond:

Option 1

Months 7 and 10: Do month 4 exercises

Months 8 and 11: Do month 5 exercises

Months 9 and 12: Do month 6 exercises

Option 2

Weeks 1, 4, 7, and 10: Do month 4 exercises

Weeks 2, 5, 8, and 11: Do month 5 exercises

Weeks 3, 6, 9, and 12: Do month 6 exercises

By changing up the exercises every four weeks or so, you keep the body challenged so you don't plateau or regress. The body seeks homeostasis, and if you keep doing the same thing over and over again, you eventually become more efficient. This results in needing less muscle to accomplish the exercises, thus you get weaker over time. To avoid this, shake things up by doing more reps or sets, or performing the exercise for a longer period of time. All of these will work. By changing your exercise program completely (by doing the past workouts), your body never gets used to the exercise program and will continue to progress. Consider the exercises given in this chapter as your foundation, your anchor. These are exercises you can return to again and again to reinforce your newfound stabilization and core strength that will help you reduce your LBP and result in a stronger body that is more resilient and resistant to injury.

If you need further help creating a workout program, I highly suggest hiring a personal trainer or Pilates instructor to design an additional program for your stronger body; one that you can follow on your own or under their watchful eye. Make sure they have some understanding or experience working with someone who has had nonspecific low back pain. I strongly suggest working with someone with a Pilates background because Pilates is such a great way to keep your core strong and body fit.

CHAPTER 8

Disc Bulge and Herniation

Spinal discs are susceptible to herniation because of the amount of mobility in the spinal segments. If we regularly exceed those ranges of motion, damage will often occur. Disc bulges and herniations are therefore some of the most common causes of low back pain. Generally they occur more often in men than women at around a two-to-one ratio[1] with the highest prevalence in the 30- to 50-year-old age group.[2] Ninety-five percent of herniations occur in the lower lumbar spine (L4 to L5, L5 to S1),[3] with the remaining five percent occurring in the cervical and thoracic spine. In this chapter, we talk specifically about lumbar disc herniations.

Definition

A disc bulge is a condition in which the outer rings of the annulus fibrosis have degraded such that the outer rings have deformed, creating what looks to be a bulge extending outward from the disc (see figure 8.1). A full herniation occurs when all the annular rings have been broken through and the nucleus is pushed out beyond the rings (see figure 8.2).

The majority of disc bulges and herniations occur in the posterior-lateral area of the disc. On a clock face, this would be at approximately five o'clock and seven o'clock, with 12 o'clock being the most anterior portion of the disc. This five o'clock and seven o'clock area is more susceptible to herniations because it doesn't have the same amount of ligament reinforcement as the anterior portion of the disc. Unfortunately, the spinal cord resides in this area, as well as the nerves coming out of the spinal cord that run peripherally throughout the body. This is an area that is overpopulated: There is way too much demand for real estate and not enough to share. This leads to those discs pushing into the nerve root resulting in pain.

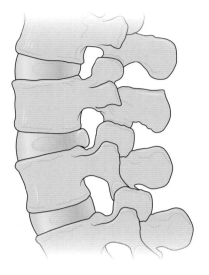

FIGURE 8.1 Disc bulge.

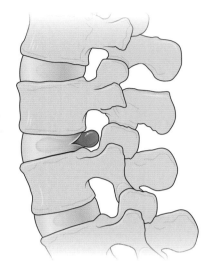

FIGURE 8.2 Disc herniation.

Straight Talk

A disc bulge is a condition with which I have personal experience. When I was in my early 20s (young, stubborn, and thought I knew everything), I hurt my back seriously. I was working as a personal trainer in my mom's personal training facility. We were getting new carpet installed and all of the equipment needed to be moved out of the current space and into another suite next door. I piled all the free weights onto a four-wheel dolly, pushed it next door, and then bent over to dump the weights off the dolly. While the exact amount of the weights is unknown, needless to say it was way beyond my capabilities. As I lifted the weight, I had the sensation of a rip cord being pulled from my butt up my spine. I stood there frozen, scared to move. But after a few seconds I did move and didn't feel too bad. However, the following morning, I couldn't walk. This is not an exaggeration. I had to crawl to the bathroom. Over the next 48 hours I had massage and chiropractic care that did wonders (being 23 years old also helped) and I didn't think anything of it. I was cured. Little did I know that this back injury was going to rear its ugly head over and over again throughout my life. This was the genesis of my back problems, and years of wear and tear have made it worse, unfortunately. My diagnosis is multilevel disc bulges. With exercise, I am able to keep most of the pain at bay, but it requires diligence and vigilance on my part to keep my bulged discs strong and stable.

Causes

For the most part, both disc bulges and herniations are accumulation injuries, meaning they take place over a long period of time. This injury rarely happens as a result of one accident or trauma, although it can occur in extreme situations like an auto accident, a fall down multiple stairs, or trying to lift far too much weight. Normally the walls of the annulus fibrosis are torn slowly over time. However, we often hear from people that there is a straw-that-broke-the-camel's-back moment, as I've previously mentioned. This moment usually involves bending over with a little bit of rotation. I tell clients in this situation that it wasn't picking up the newspaper or pencil that blew out their back, but the thousands of repetitions that preceded it. Other risk factors can include smoking, heavy weight-bearing activities such as weightlifting, and certain work-related movements such as repetitive lifting.[4]

Symptoms

The symptoms of a disc bulge and a herniation are similar and fairly easy to identify. Numbness and tingling down the leg are one of the first symptoms; radiating pain down the leg (radiculopathy) is another. These symptoms develop as a result of nerve compression or irritation. Bulges and herniations can compress the nerve root, which sends the signals down the leg. If you've ever had your foot fall asleep, that sensation is similar to the numbness or tingling you may feel with a disc injury. It can range from mildly annoying to incredibly irritating because it never seems to go away. This happened to me after demonstrating an exercise to a client without being properly warmed up. For the next week, I had numbness in the toes of my right foot that would not go away. It was extremely annoying and I found it hard to concentrate on anything else.

Referred pain and radiating pain signals are also common symptoms of a disc bulge or herniation. Referred pain is felt in an area other than the injury, while radiating pain starts in one area and spreads down the limb, and in the case of disc injuries, usually the leg. I've had a number of clients whose pain was minimal in their back but more pronounced in their thigh or the inside of the knee.

Straight Talk

An interesting fact is that 19 to 27 percent of people exhibiting no low back pain are discovered to have disc herniations upon MRI.[5] Anyone who has low back pain may wonder how is that is possible, but if the protrusion doesn't press on and irritate a nerve, there is no pain. The protruded disc matter could be less than a millimeter away from the nerve, but so long as there is no contact, there is no pain.

There are various medical muscle tests that can help to diagnose a herniated or bulging disc; however, the only precise diagnosis is with an MRI, which will accurately indicate the problem and its location. It can indicate a slight bulge, full herniation, or anything in between. Be leery of someone who claims to know exactly what is wrong without doing any further imaging—a herniation can't be seen with an X-ray. It can be suspected, but the MRI will speak the truth.

Treatment Options

Depending on how conservative the doctor is, treatment options range from rest, ice, and anti-inflammatories to physical therapy and eventually surgery. The choice will be up to you and your doctor based on what has been discovered. With good physical therapy, the outcomes can not only be positive, but there can often be full recovery. However, there are cases where surgery is necessary. If your doctor indicates that surgery is necessary, I suggest getting multiple opinions, especially if you are given other treatment options. Some improvement through very conservative treatments is the norm, with only about 10 percent of people still having sufficient pain after six weeks to contemplate surgery. In fact, follow-up MRIs have shown that the herniated or bulging portion of the disc tends to regress over time, and two-thirds of patients have partial to complete resolution after six months.[6]

Physical therapy is a helpful and very common prescription, typically suggested before a physician does surgery. Ideally, physical therapy will reduce inflammation, relax muscle spasms, and reeducate core and spinal stabilizers. Much of what you read about in this and other chapters builds on knowledge gained from participating in physical therapy; however, this text is not designed to replace it. Physical therapy can do a world of good. I highly recommend you take advantage of it and then follow up with these exercises. A good physical therapist will teach you about proper body positioning during exercise, correct lifting mechanics, and appropriate work and home ergonomics, all specific to your disc herniation or bulge. A great therapist will set you up to successfully manage your condition.

Contraindications

Toward the end of chapter one, we introduced the concept of directional preference or pelvic bias. Certain exercises are going to be contraindicated for you if you have a disc herniation or bulge. You need to make sure you are doing the correct exercises to achieve your goals as quickly as possible. If you have a disc bulge or herniation, the primary contraindication is spinal flexion. You really need to avoid this at all costs. Spinal flexion will put pressure on your lumbar discs and will increase the amount of pressure on the nerve root from the disc bulge or herniation.

You need to be in a *spinal extension bias* (refer back to figure 1.6*b* on page 18 for an example), which means that your back should always have an arch to it. Remember when we talked about the pelvis tipping forward or backward? If it were a bowl filled with water, an extension bias would put you into an anterior pelvic tilt, meaning if you arched your back your pelvis would tip forward and the water would pour out in front of your body (see figure 8.3). This pushes the disc material forward as you arch your back, which takes pressure off the nerve root and can actually decompress the nerve root entirely. Many people with disc bulges or herniations find relief when they stand, lean back, and arch their low back. In fact, this is one of the famous McKenzie exercises often prescribed after someone is diagnosed. The McKenzie exercises were developed by Robin McKenzie, a physical therapist from New Zealand in 1981.[7] The common exercises developed by McKenzie involve doing exercises that put the body in spinal extension, or extension bias. A recent study evaluated the effectiveness of the McKenzie method compared to manual therapy in managing chronic low back pain and concluded that the McKenzie method is a successful treatment to decrease pain in the short term and enhance function in the long term.[8] Many of the exercises suggested in this chapter will be in extension bias position. When lying on your back you want to make sure you DO NOT flatten your back! You need to have an arch in it.

I had a client with such severe back pain caused by a disc herniation that she thought she would never be out of pain. By doing the correct exercises with an extension bias she was able to achieve 95 percent relief. Even so, certain activities, like gardening, cause her back to flare up so she has to be conscientious about her position while doing activities that include a lot of bending and forward flexing. These positions are the exact opposite of those that make her back feel better. Even sitting in her husband's low-slung car can put her into too much flexion and irritate her back. She needs to be kept in an extension bias in order to avoid pain. This requires her to modify how she moves when getting in and out of cars and gardening. She must focus on maintaining an arch in her back during all activities.

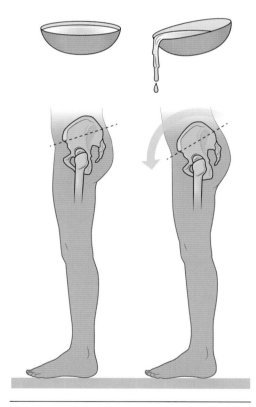

FIGURE 8.3 Visualizing your pelvis as a bowl of water in which the water spills to the front when in anterior pelvic tilt.

When performing these exercises, keep your neutral spine arched with that extension bias. Regardless of whether you are lying down, seated, or standing, a neutral spine will keep an arch in your low back.

Training Focus

The following exercise programs described in tables 8.1 through 8.6 will help to manage your bulge or herniation. Each month, you will either add new exercises or replace some of your current exercises with more advanced ones. The goal is progression: You want to move forward, and the only way to do that is to work a little harder by adjusting one of the variables. Those variables are volume (the number of sets and repetitions, or total number of exercises), load (the amount of weight being lifted), and frequency (the number of exercise days per week). Each month, you can look forward to a change in your exercise program, and as long as you are not experiencing increased pain, you will continue with the new exercise program until the next month. If you have increased pain, go back to the previous month for another week or two, then give the new exercise program another try.

Keep in mind that not all exercises are meant for everybody. There may be an exercise that works for one person but may cause someone else significant discomfort. Simply avoid any exercise that hurts. Come back to that exercise later in the month or even the following month to see if you have become strong enough to do it without pain. From my personal and professional experience, I know there may be an exercise that you will never be able to do, and that's okay. If you can not perform this one exercise, it will not make or break your success. Do the exercises that don't cause you pain and avoid the ones that do.

Sometimes, however, mild discomfort is a sign that you're stretching and flexing beyond your previous ability. What kind of pain is okay and what kind is not? Normally we instruct our clients that a little discomfort is all right. On a scale of 1 to 10, with 1 being no pain at all and a 10 being the worst pain you can imagine, where would you rank your pain as you perform an exercise? If it is at a 1 to a 3, it is okay to work through it. This would include some mild discomfort. However, if the pain is severe, don't perform the exercise that day. You may feel some pain with the first or second repetition of an exercise and want to immediately stop. I encourage you to do a couple more repetitions and see if the pain dissipates. It often will. However, if the pain continues above level 3, don't push through. Let it go for the day, and move on to the next exercise. And if every exercise is causing discomfort beyond a level 3, then lay off the exercises for a day or two. Let things calm down before trying them again. If the pain persists, please contact your physician.

You will begin by getting comfortable with the exercises and establishing the habit of doing them regularly. I often tell my clients to do the exercises every day. It sounds like a lot but let's face reality: Most people will do the exercises three to four times per week. That's perfect. However, when I tell them to do it three to four times per week, they may actually do it only once or twice. Success hinges on your consistency. The more you do the exercises, the stronger you will get.

Before You Begin: Finding Neutral Spine and Engaging Kegels

Neutral spine was first discussed in detail back in chapter 1, but it is worth repeating because it applies specifically to your bulging or herniated disc and the exercises prescribed in the following program. When talking about low back pain, neutral spine is the spinal position you can maintain with little to no pain. The following exercises should be performed in a pain-free neutral spine.

The clinical definition of *neutral spine* is the position in which the anterior superior iliac spine is on the same plane as the posterior superior iliac spine. While those anatomical landmarks mean something to many health care professionals, they don't translate nearly as well to the general population. For the rest of us, neutral spine is the position in which your spine has the least amount of stress on it, where the curves of the cervical, thoracic, and lumbar regions support each other and are able to cushion the spine optimally. We will focus primarily on the lumbar spine, but remember that if you change the angle of one region, the others will also change. For someone with a bulging or herniated disc, the pelvis should be in an anterior tilt (extension bias), so having a larger arch to the spine would not be uncommon and will probably feel better and be less painful. This position with a larger arch would be considered your neutral spine.

You may have multiple conditions you are managing along with your herniation or bulge, and being in an extension bias may cause pain or discomfort. Don't force yourself into a painful posture. If you also have stenosis or spondylolisthesis then you should read those specific chapters before proceeding. Chances are that you may feel better in a slight posterior pelvic tilt (a flatter back posture). The exercises in those chapters may be safer for you to do. Listen to your body. If a slightly flattened to fully flattened back feels better, then do the exercises in the chapter that corresponds to your other condition.

You will see that the first exercise in month 1 is to find your neutral spine and maintain it. Lie down (supine) on your back in a position that produces little to no pain, or such that the pain subsides as you continue to relax on your back. Next, find your Kegel muscles. These are usually described as the muscles that help to hold back a stream of urine. They are your pelvic floor muscles, a muscle group that comprises part of your inner core, and they should be slightly engaged during these exercises. Don't grip them hard, just a light hold: think 30 percent of your maximum. Hold for about 20 to 30 seconds. As you become stronger, it will become easier to maintain. Focus on keeping the muscles engaged throughout each exercise. It may not be easy, and you may forget. Once you can find neutral spine and engage the pelvic floor muscles, it's time to move on to the exercises.

Table 8.1   Month 1 Exercises

1. Neutral spine and Kegel		Hold for 30 sec	
2. Bent-knee fallout		2 sets of 10 reps each side	Page 55
3. Heel slide		2 sets of 10 reps each side (alternating)	Page 56
4. Marching		2 sets of 10 reps each side (alternating)	Page 57
5. Pelvic press hold		10 sec hold for 5 reps	Page 70
6. Pelvic press hip extension		1 sec hold for 2 sets of 10 reps each side (alternating)	Page 71
7. Kneeling hip flexor stretch		30 sec hold for 2 sets each side	Page 111
8. Doorway hamstring stretch		60 sec hold for 2 sets each side	Page 112

Table 8.2   Month 2 Exercises

1. Bent-knee fallout		2 sets of 20 reps each side	Page 55
2. Marching		2 sets of 20 reps each side (alternating)	Page 57
3. March-up		2 sets of 10 reps each side (alternating)	Page 58
4. Leg lowering		2 sets of 10 reps each side (alternating)	Page 59
5. Straight-back bridge		2 sets of 10 reps	Page 64
6. Pelvic press hip extension		1 sec hold for 2 sets of 10 reps each side (alternating)	Page 71
7. Pelvic press shoulder retraction		5 reps of 5 sec hold for 2 sets	Page 72
8. Kneeling hip flexor stretch		30 sec hold for 2 sets each side	Page 111
9. Doorway hamstring stretch		60 sec hold for 2 sets each side	Page 112

Table 8.3   Month 3 Exercises

Exercise		Reps	Page
1. March-up		2 sets of 20 reps each side (alternating)	Page 58
2. Leg lowering		2 sets of 20 reps each side (alternating)	Page 59
3. Dying bug		2 sets of 20 reps each side	Page 61
4. Advanced kick-out		2 sets of 8 reps each side	Page 60
5. Straight-back bridge		2 sets of 20 reps	Page 64
6. Quadruped hip extension lift		2 sets of 10 reps each side	Page 79
7. Quadruped birddog		2 sets of 10 reps each side	Page 80
8. Kneeling hip flexor stretch		30 sec hold for 2 sets each side	Page 111
9. Strap hamstring stretch		60 sec hold for 2 sets each side	Page 113

Table 8.4   Month 4 Exercises

1. Dying bug		2 sets of 20 reps each side	Page 61
2. Advanced kick-out		2 sets of 12 reps each side	Page 60
3. Straight-back bridge		2 sets of 20 reps	Page 64
4. Stability ball hip extension hold		5 reps of 10 sec hold for 2 sets. Focus on a small range of motion, and do not arch the back.	Page 90
5. Ball birddog		2 sets of 8 reps each side. Stay in a posterior tilt.	Page 91
6. Tube press-out		2 sets of 12 reps each side	Page 93
7. Tube circle		2 sets of 12 reps each side in both directions	Page 94

(Continued)

Table 8.4   Month 4 Exercises *(continued)*

8. High plank		10 sec hold for 2 sets, working up to 30 sec hold	Page 81
9. Standing telescope arms		8 reps each side	Page 105
10. Kneeling hip flexor stretch		30 sec hold for 2 sets each side	Page 111
11. Strap hamstring stretch		60 sec hold for 2 sets each side	Page 113

Table 8.5 Month 5 Exercises

1. Tube press-out		2 sets of 12 reps each side	Page 93
2. Tube circle		2 sets of 12 reps each side in both directions	Page 94
3. Tube walk-out		2 sets of 5 reps each side	Page 95
4. Full plank		3 reps of 10 sec hold for 2 sets with 10 sec rest between reps	Page 82
5. Stability ball hip extension hold		5 reps of 10 sec hold for 2 sets each side. Focus on a small range of motion, and do not arch the back.	Page 90
6. Ball birddog		2 sets of 8 reps each side. Do not arch the back.	Page 91

(Continued)

Table 8.5 Month 5 Exercises (continued)

7. Stand-up–sit-down		2 sets of 30 reps	Page 99
8. Clock step		2 sets of 5 reps each direction (12, 2, & 3 o'clock; then 12, 10, & 9 o'clock)	Page 98
9. Standing telescope arms		2 sets of 8 reps each side	Page 105
10. Kneeling hip flexor stretch		30 sec hold for 2 sets each side	Page 111
11. Strap hamstring stretch		60 sec hold for 2 sets each side	Page 113

Table 8.6   Month 6 Exercises

1. Tube press-out		2 sets of 12 reps each side	Page 93
2. Tube circle		2 sets of 12 reps each side in both directions	Page 94
3. Tube walk-out		2 sets of 5 reps each side	Page 95
4. Full plank		5 reps of 10 sec hold for 2 sets with 3 sec rest between reps	Page 82
5. Chicken wing		1 set of 12 reps each side	page 106

(Continued)

Table 8.6   Month 6 Exercises *(continued)*

6. Tube single-arm row		5 reps of 10 sec hold for 2 sets each side	Page 96
7. Tube single-arm press		2 sets of 8 reps each side	Page 97
8. Stand-up–sit-down		2 sets of 30 reps	Page 99
9. Clock step		2 sets of 5 reps each direction (12, 2, & 3 o'clock; then 12, 10, & 9 o'clock)	Page 98
10. Kneeling hip flexor stretch		30 sec hold for 2 reps each side	Page 111
11. Strap hamstring stretch		60 sec hold for 2 reps each side	Page 113

Continuing Your Training

By the end of the sixth month, you should be able to include general weight training in your exercise program. The trick is to not ask too much of your body too quickly, so start small using lighter weights and work your way up. I highly recommend the use of machines in this phase of training because they are a relatively safe way to get back into lifting weights. Machines put you in a dedicated path of motion, which eliminates some of the inherent instability of free weights. This may go against what some trainers have told you in the past, but you are now reintroducing your body to weight training and if you ask too much of your body, it may fail and send you backward. Keep in mind that this is temporary; as you become stronger, you can reintroduce free weights to your exercise program. This will challenge you to stabilize in many different planes of motion and will be an important part of strength building once you're ready.

With each exercise, especially seated exercises, you need to make sure that you are keeping a bit more arch your spine because you have a disc bulge or herniation. Focus on keeping the extension bias in your spine. You need to make sure that when you sit, you don't tuck your tailbone and flatten your back. Keep an arch in your back throughout the exercises.

I realize, too, that not everyone belongs to a gym. In that case, you can continue to do month 5 exercises indefinitely. But remember that the body gets used to what it does regularly and will stagnate and weaken over time if you don't change things up a bit. You can always increase reps, sets, or even hold times to jazz it up a bit. To challenge your body, I suggest one of the following two options for month 7 and beyond:

Option 1

    Months 7 and 10: Do month 4 exercises

    Months 8 and 11: Do month 5 exercises

    Months 9 and 12: Do month 6 exercises

Option 2

    Weeks 1, 4, 7, and 10: Do month 4 exercises

    Weeks 2, 5, 8, and 11: Do month 5 exercises

    Weeks 3, 6, 9, and 12: Do month 6 exercises

By changing up the exercises every four weeks or so, you keep the body challenged so you don't plateau. The body seeks homeostasis, and if you keep doing the same thing over and over again, you eventually become more efficient. This results in needing less muscle to accomplish the exercises, thus you get weaker over time. To avoid this, shake things up by doing more reps or sets, or performing the exercise for a longer period of time. All of these will work. By changing your exercise program completely (by doing the past workouts), your body never gets used to the routine and will continue to progress. As you progress, you will likely experience a slow decrease in pain and discomfort as you become stronger. Your symptoms will lessen in severity and hopefully diminish over time. Remember your goal is to become stable in your spine, and as you become increasingly more stable, you will find yourself becoming more functional as well.

If you need further help creating a workout program, I suggest hiring a personal trainer to design a program that you can follow on your own. Make sure they have some understanding in working with someone who has had a disc bulge or herniation. I also highly recommend working with someone with a Pilates background. Pilates is a great way to keep your core strong and your body fit, and many Pilates instructors have experience working with people with disc bulges and herniations.

CHAPTER 9

Spondylolisthesis

Spondylolisthesis is a spinal condition in which one vertebra slips off another, most often in the lumbosacral region between the L4 and L5 vertebrae. It is rarely seen in people under the age of 50 because degeneration seems to be a primary cause of the condition. Women are about five times more likely than men to have spondylolisthesis.[1] Spondylolisthesis is the condition that most people neglect to mention when relaying their MRI results to me. Why? Many times, they don't know what it is, they can't pronounce it, and therefore, they forget about it.

Definition

The etymology of the word *spondylolisthesis* comes from the Greek word for dislocation or slipping. This means that in a particular spinal segment (two vertebrae and the disc in between), the top vertebra has slipped off the bottom one. The most common version of this is called an anterolisthesis, where the top vertebra have slipped anteriorly over the bottom one (see figure 9.1). If you think about the natural lordosis (curve) to the lumbar spine, the bodies of the vertebrae angle downward in the lower portion of the lumbar spine. Gravity is constantly pulling on them and one theory shows a correlation between a higher body mass index and the development of spondylolisthesis in females.[2] More research is needed, but increased spinal loading may be a contributing factor to anterolisthesis.[3]

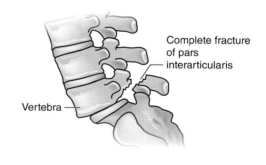

FIGURE 9.1 Anterolisthesis of the spine, which is a common version of spondylolisthesis.

Spondylolisthesis is often diagnosed with a "grade" indicating the degree of slippage in order to classify its severity. Grades I through V are classified as follows:

- *Grade I:* 1 to 25 percent slip
- *Grade II:* 26 to 50 percent slip
- *Grade III:* 51 to 75 percent slip
- *Grade IV:* 76 to 100 percent slip
- *Grade V:* Complete dislocation, greater than 100 percent

According to the Cleveland Clinic, grade I and grade II slips usually don't require surgical intervention and a more conservative approach to treatment is considered first. However, grades III and IV, and especially grade V, may require surgery if pain remains persistent and function is compromised.[4]

Causes

The two most common forms of spondylolisthesis are traumatic and degenerative. Traumatic spondylolisthesis is a result of an acute traumatic injury involving either bony or soft tissue posterior spinal elements accompanied with slippage of one vertebral body over another.[5] In other words, some type of trauma struck the spine with such force that there is a slippage of one vertebra over another. Most often this occurs during traffic accidents and serious falls—an event that places a lot of shearing force on the body and especially the spine. The most common area of occurrence is at the very bottom of the spine at L5 to S1, the lumbosacral junction. This type of spondylolisthesis is often accompanied by a spinal fracture in the area leading to the instability that causes the slippage.

A second type of spondylolisthesis—the most common type—is degenerative. This is most often age-related and caused by the accumulation of a lifetime of spinal stresses resulting in the degeneration of the disc and spine. We usually see this type of spondylolisthesis at L4 to L5. Believe it or not, this form of spondylolisthesis is often fairly stable and patients can have it for a long time without knowing until something triggers the low back pain. Interestingly, the greater the degeneration in the disc—meaning, the less disc height you have—the more stable the area. One hypothesis is that the degenerative process acts with "self-limiting inhibitory control on further slip progression."[6] The more degenerated the disc, the less slippage there is. However, this doesn't mean that the person will have no pain. In chapter 10, we'll discuss stenosis, a condition in which the disc degenerates and the disc space narrows, causing pain.

Straight Talk

I have a client who initially came to me with fairly severe low back pain caused by the degenerative form of spondylolisthesis. Over time, he became stronger and was relatively pain-free in his back. It appears that part of the reason for his decreased pain is that the degeneration in his back advanced to the point that it most likely fused itself in a pain-free position. This is one potential outcome of the degeneration process. However, it doesn't always end this way: His back could just as easily have fused in a way that compressed the nerve instead, and that would have caused him greater discomfort and pain. Whether it was luck of the draw or the fact that he was diligent with his exercises and with keeping his pelvis in proper position, we will never know. But he is thankful that we've been able to keep him strong and stable throughout the years.

Symptoms

The primary symptom for traumatic spondylolisthesis is pain. Approximately half of those with spondylolisthesis are also affected by a neurologic issue, whether it is motor (involving muscle) or sensory (numbness, tingling, or radiating pain), often caused by the compression of the nerve root in the foramen exiting the spine.[7] The symptoms we often see with degenerative spondylolisthesis is generalized lower back pain or spasm, muscle cramping, numbness, tingling, or radiculopathy pain down the leg. These symptoms can be intermittent or constant.

Spondylolisthesis is usually diagnosed with an X-ray, but an MRI will show much greater detail and provide a better picture of what is actually happening with the nerves and tissues.

Treatment Options

Conservative, nonsurgical treatments are often the first course of action. These may include an anti-inflammatory medication (NSAID), epidural or steroidal injections, and physical therapy. The NSAIDS and epidurals help to reduce the inflammation and calm the area down. Physical therapy reeducates and wakes up the muscles to allow them to stabilize the spine better, which is precisely what you will be doing with your exercises. Again, these exercises do not take the place of physical therapy, but can enhance and build upon what you have learned during a course of physical therapy.

For the most part, patients should only consider surgery when conservative options have been exhausted. Surgery will often be a type of laminectomy or a spinal fusion (see chapter 11 for more information about spinal surgeries). A laminectomy will help decompress the nerves, while the fusion will stabilize the joint by fixating it in place. A spinal fusion can be done many different ways, and your physician will typically determine the method based on the severity of the case. This is a very serious surgery—as drastic as a joint replacement—and should not be taken lightly. The spinal structure is forever changed by replacing the disc with a man-made object.

However, not all cases of spondylolisthesis result in pain. Remember, if the instability isn't great enough to cause any nerve compression then there may not be any resultant pain from this condition. If you have this diagnosis, however, you will still benefit from the exercises in this section—the fact that you don't currently have pain doesn't mean you never will. Think of it as preventative maintenance. A Chinese proverb says, "The best time to plant a tree was 20 years ago. The second-best time is now." I can't tell you how many clients wish they had started years ago, before the pain got bad.

Contraindications

When I see spondylolisthesis documented on someone's MRI, a red flag goes up in my mind because this condition will dictate the client's pelvic bias and has some of the strictest contraindications. Anyone with spondylolisthesis needs to be kept in a posterior pelvic tilt, meaning that your pelvic "bowl" needs to be tipped so that if it were holding water, the water would tilt out

the back of the bowl (see figure 9.2). Another way of thinking about it is if you are lying down you would want to flatten your back to the floor by tucking your pelvis.

Think of your pelvis as the face of a clock with 6 o'clock being at the belly button and 12 o'clock being between the thighs (see figure 9.3). At the center of the clock where the hands rotate around, imagine there is a marble. Tuck your pelvis such that the marble will roll toward 6 o'clock. Then return it back to the center of the clock. DO NOT tilt your pelvis the other direction! That's where danger lies. Your happy place will be with your tail tucked and your back flattened out.

The main contraindication is arching the back. Don't do it! If you keep your pelvis tilted posteriorly you will keep your back and spine safe. You will work on how to do this in the exercises given. The progression of exercises is as follows: lying on your

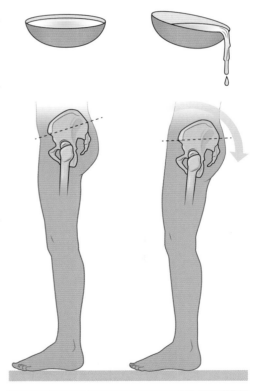

FIGURE 9.2 Visualizing the pelvis as a bowl of water in which the water spills to the back in a posterior pelvic tilt.

back in the supine position, lying prone on your stomach, being on all fours, being seated, and finally standing.

I do realize that standing and walking around with a posterior tilt conjures up the visual of an old man with his belt pulled up under his chest, but that is the extreme. We want your spine a little flatter and your pelvis slightly tucked under. What you might feel in your spine is a softening of your back. It will be a slight stretch for these muscles, especially if you are a person who has a pretty large lordosis, or curve to the spine. Those spinal muscles are under constant

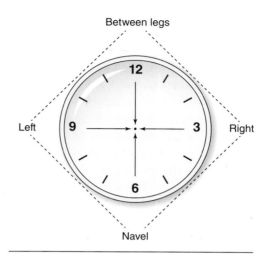

FIGURE 9.3 Visualize your pelvis as a clock face to find your optimum 6 o'clock pelvic position.

tension, remaining in a shortened position all the time. We want them to be softened and supple, even relaxed. But this will take time. Have patience: These muscles may have been under this continuous tension for many years. It may take time to reverse years of muscle memory.

Training Focus

The following exercise programs described in tables 9.1 through 9.6 will help to manage your spondylolisthesis. Each month, you will either add new exercises or replace some of your current exercises with more advanced ones. The goal is progression: You want to move forward, and the only way to do that is to work a little harder by adjusting one of the variables. Those variables are volume (the number of sets and repetitions, or total number of exercises), load (the amount of weight being lifted), and frequency (the number of exercise days per week). Each month, you can look forward to a change in your exercise program, and as long as you are not experiencing increased pain, you will continue with the new exercise program until the next month. If you have increased pain, go back to the previous month for another week or two, then give the new exercise program another try.

Keep in mind that not all exercises are meant for everybody. There may be an exercise that works for one person but may cause another person significant discomfort. Simply avoid any exercise that hurts. Come back to that exercise later in the month or even the following month to see if you have become strong enough to do it without pain. From my personal and professional experience, I know there may be an exercise that you will never be able to do, and that's okay. If you can not perform this one exercise, it will not make or break your success. Do the ones that don't cause you pain and avoid the ones that do.

Let's discuss what kind of pain is okay and what kind is not. Normally we instruct our clients that a little discomfort is all right. On a scale of 1 to 10, with 1 being no pain at all and a 10 being the worst pain you can imagine, where would you rank your pain as you perform an exercise? If it is at a 1 to a 3, it is okay to work through it. This would include some mild discomfort. However, if the pain is severe, don't perform the exercise that day. You may feel some pain with the first or second repetition of an exercise, and want to immediately stop. I encourage you to do a couple more repetitions and see if the pain dissipates. It often will. However, if the pain continues above level 3, don't push through. Let it go for the day, and move on to the next exercise. If every exercise is causing discomfort beyond a level 3, then lay off the exercises for a day or two. Let things calm down before trying them again. If the pain persists, please contact your physician.

You will begin by getting comfortable with the exercises and establishing the habit of doing them regularly. I often tell my clients to do the exercises every day. It sounds like a lot but let's face reality: Most people will do the exercises three to four times per week. That's perfect. However, when I tell them to do it three to four times per week, they may actually do it only once or twice. Success hinges on your consistency. The more you do the exercises, the stronger you will get.

For the first few exercises, I suggest using a Togu Pilates balance ball. I particularly like this ball because it has great tactile feedback; it is strong enough to lie on but still has some springiness to it. Regular beach balls are also a possibility; if that's what you use, I recommend a 20-inch size for most people. The beach ball is an economical option, however it won't provide the same tactile feedback as the Togu ball. Also, we will be using the Togu ball mostly deflated, about 20 to 25 percent full. I put in two big breaths when I am inflating it. Start there and see how it feels. If it feels too big, like you are too high up in the air, let some air out. You know you need more air in it if the ball bottoms out when you get on it.

Lie down with the Togu ball under your pelvis, not your low back. It should be under your sacrum, and your sacrum should be level. To find this position, I recommend laying down with the ball under your back, sitting up, and then wedging the ball under your rear end as far as you can. Once you do this, slowly curl your body down onto your back with your feet remaining on the floor and knees at approximately 90 degrees. You will know it is too high (toward your low back) if you feel as though the ball is trying to arch your back. Likewise, it is too low if it places you into a tucked position. Between the two, being slightly too low is preferable to being slightly too high, especially with spondylolisthesis.

Before You Begin: Finding Neutral Spine and Engaging Kegels

Neutral spine was first discussed in detail back in chapter 1, but it is worth repeating because it applies specifically to spondylolisthesis and the exercises prescribed in the following program. When talking about low back pain, neutral spine is the spinal position you can maintain with little to no pain. The exercises should be performed in your pain-free neutral spine.

The clinical definition of *neutral spine* is the position in which the anterior superior iliac spine is on the same plane as the posterior superior iliac spine. While those anatomical landmarks mean something to many health care professionals, they don't translate nearly as well to the general population. For the rest of us, neutral spine is the position in which your spine has the least amount of stress on it, where the curves of the cervical, thoracic and lumbar regions support each other and are able to cushion the spine optimally. We will focus primarily on the lumbar spine, but remember that if you change the angle of one region, the others will also change, for better or worse. For someone with spondylolisthesis, the spine and pelvis need to be in a flexion bias, with the lumbar spine being flexed and the pelvis being in a posterior tilt (refer back to figure 9.2 on page 164). In the supine position this would mean lying with a flat back and the pelvis tucked under. To achieve this flat back posture in a prone position, I suggest using a pillow or two under your stomach, as this will allow the spine to stay flexed.

You will see that the first exercise in month 1 is to find your neutral spine and maintain it. Lie down (supine) on your back in a position that produces little to no pain, or such that the pain subsides as you continue to relax on your back. Next, find your Kegel muscles. These are usually described as the muscles that help to hold back a stream of urine. They are your pelvic floor muscles, a muscle group that comprises part of your inner core, and they should be slightly engaged during these exercises. Don't grip them hard, just a light hold: think 30 percent of your maximum. Hold for about 20 to 30 seconds. As you become stronger, it will become easier to maintain. Focus on keeping the muscles engaged throughout each exercise. It may not be easy, and you may forget. Once you can find neutral spine and engage the pelvic floor muscles, it's time to move on to the exercises.

Table 9.1   Month 1 Exercises

1. Neutral spine and Kegel		Hold for 30 sec	
2. Togu pelvic tilt (with hold)		5 reps of 5 sec hold for 2 sets	Page 65
3. Togu pelvic tilt		2 sets of 10 reps	Page 65
4. Togu marching		2 sets of 10 reps each side (alternating)	Page 66
5. Lying lumbar stretch		30 sec hold for 2 sets	Page 114
6. Heel slide		2 sets of 10 reps each side. For spondylolisthesis, perform with a flattened back; do not let the back arch as the leg is extended.	Page 56
7. Bent-knee fallout		2 sets of 10 reps each side. For spondylolisthesis, perform with a flattened back.	Page 55
8. Cat and cow		2 sets of 10 reps. For spondylolisthesis, focus only on the rounding of the back; do not arch the back.	Page 103

Table 9.1   Month 1 Exercises

9. Doorway hamstring stretch		60 sec hold for 2 sets. For spondylolisthesis, keep the opposite knee bent and the back flat.	Page 112
10. Knee-to-chest stretch		30 sec hold for 2 reps each side	Page 116

Table 9.2   Month 2 Exercises

1. Togu pelvic tilt		2 sets of 20 reps	Page 65
2. Togu marching		2 sets of 10 reps each side (alternating)	Page 66
3. Togu tilted march-up		2 sets of 8 reps each side (alternating)	Page 67
4. Togu leg lowering with pelvic tilt		2 sets of 8 reps each side (alternating)	Page 68
5. Lying lumbar stretch		30 sec hold for 2 sets	Page 114

(Continued)

Table 9.2   Month 2 Exercises *(continued)*

6. Heel slide		2 sets of 20 reps each side	Page 56
7. Lying overhead reach		2 sets of 10 reps each side	Page 63
8. Dying bug		2 sets of 8 reps each side. For spondylolisthesis, perform with a flat back.	Page 61
9. Strap hamstring stretch		30 sec hold for 2 sets each side. For spondylolisthesis, keep the opposite knee bent and the back flat.	Page 113
10. Knee-to-chest stretch		30 sec hold for 2 reps each side	Page 116
11. Seated lumbar stretch		30 sec hold for 2 reps	Page 115

Table 9.3 Month 3 Exercises

1. Togu pelvic tilt		2 sets of 20 reps.	Page 65
2. Togu tilted march-up		2 sets of 8 reps each side (alternating)	Page 67
3. Togu leg lowering with pelvic tilt		2 sets of 8 reps each side (alternating)	Page 68
4. Lying lumbar stretch		30 sec hold for 2 sets	Page 114
5. Dying bug		2 sets of 12 reps each side. For spondylolisthesis, perform with a flat back.	Page 61
6. Articulating bridge		2 sets of 12 reps. For spondylolisthesis, focus on the pelvic tilt.	Page 108
7. Pelvic press hold		5 sec hold for 5 reps. For spondylolisthesis, place a pillow under the stomach and allow a posterior tilt of the pelvis.	Page 70

(Continued)

Table 9.3   Month 3 Exercises *(continued)*

Exercise	Image	Sets/Reps	Page
8. Pelvic press hip extension		2 sets of 8 reps each side. For spondylolisthesis, place a pillow under the stomach, allow posterior tilt of the pelvis, and focus on a small range of motion.	Page 71
9. Quadruped hold with opposite-arm tap		2 sets of 12 reps each side	Page 77
10. Quadruped hip extension slide		2 sets of 8 reps each side. For spondylolisthesis, keep slightly tucked under throughout; do not arch the back.	Page 78
11. Kneeling hip flexor stretch		30 sec hold for 2 sets each side. For spondylolisthesis, perform with a posterior tilt; do not arch the back.	Page 111
12. Strap hamstring stretch		60 sec hold for 2 sets each side	Page 113
13. Seated lumbar stretch		30 sec hold for 2 reps	Page 115

Table 9.4 Month 4 Exercises

1. Togu pelvic tilt		1 set of 20 reps	Page 65
2. Togu tilted march-up		2 sets of 8 reps each side (alternating)	Page 67
3. Togu leg lowering with pelvic tilt		2 sets of 8 reps each side (alternating)	Page 68
4. Lying lumbar stretch		30 sec hold for 2 sets	Page 114
5. Dying bug		2 sets of 12 reps each side. For spondylolisthesis, perform with a flat back.	Page 61
6. Articulating bridge		2 sets of 12 reps. For spondylolisthesis, focus on the pelvic tilt.	Page 108
7. Pelvic press hip extension		2 sets of 8 reps each side. For spondylolisthesis, place a pillow under the stomach, allow a posterior tilt of the pelvis, and focus on a small range of motion.	Page 71

(Continued)

Table 9.4   Month 4 Exercises *(continued)*

8. Stability ball seated hip shift		2 sets of 20 reps. For spondylolisthesis, perform side to side only.	Page 87
9. Stability ball seated knee lift		2 sets of 8 reps each side	Page 88
10. Stability ball walk-out		2 sets of 8 reps. Begin walk-out with posterior tilt.	Page 89
11. Stability ball hip extension hold		5 reps of 5 sec hold for 2 sets each side .For stenosis, keep a posterior tilt of the pelvis, focus on a small range of motion, and do not arch the back.	Page 90
12. Stand-up–sit-down		2 sets of 25 reps. For spondylolisthesis, be sure to land gently.	Page 99

Table 9.4   Month 4 Exercises

13. Kneeling hip flexor stretch		30 sec hold for 2 reps each side. For spondylolisthesis, perform with a posterior tilt; do not arch the back.	Page 111
14. Strap hamstring stretch		60 sec hold for 2 sets each side	Page 113
15. Seated lumbar stretch		30 sec hold for 2 reps	Page 115

Table 9.5   Month 5 Exercises

1. Togu pelvic tilt		1 set of 20 reps	Page 65
2. Togu tilted march-up		2 sets of 8 reps each side (alternating)	Page 67
3. Togu leg lowering with pelvic tilt		2 sets of 8 reps each side (alternating)	Page 68

(Continued)

Table 9.5 Month 5 Exercises *(continued)*

4. Lying lumbar stretch		30 sec hold for 2 reps	Page 114
5. Articulating bridge		2 sets of 12 reps. For spon- dylolisthesis, focus on the pelvic tilt.	Page 108
6. Full plank		3 reps of 10 sec hold for 2 sets with 3 sec rest between reps	Page 82
7. Stability ball walk-out		2 sets of 8 reps. Begin walk-out with posterior tilt.	Page 89
8. Stability ball hip extension hold		5 reps of 10 sec hold for 2 sets each side. For stenosis, keep a posterior tilt of the pelvis, focus on a small range of motion, and do not arch the back.	Page 90
9. Tube press-out		2 sets of 12 reps each side	Page 93

Table 9.5   Month 5 Exercises

10. Tube circle		2 sets of 8 reps each side in both directions	Page 94
11. Clock step		2 sets of 4 reps each side (12, 2, & 3 o'clock; then 12, 10, & 9 o'clock)	Page 98
12. Stand-up–sit-down		2 sets of 40 reps. For spondylolisthesis, be sure to land gently.	Page 99
13. Kneeling hip flexor stretch		30 sec hold for 2 reps each side. For spondylolisthesis, perform with a posterior tilt; do not arch the back.	Page 111
14. Strap hamstring stretch		60 sec hold for 2 sets each side	Page 113

Table 9.6   Month 6 Exercises

1. Togu pelvic tilt		1 set of 20 reps	Page 65
2. Togu tilted march-up		2 sets of 8 reps each side (alternating)	Page 67
3. Togu leg lowering with pelvic tilt		2 sets of 8 reps each side (alternating)	Page 68
4. Lying lumbar stretch		30 sec hold for 2 reps	Page 114
5. Articulating bridge		2 sets of 12 reps. For spondylolisthesis, focus on the pelvic tilt.	Page 108
6. Full plank		3 reps of 10 sec hold for 2 sets with 3 sec rest between reps	Page 82
7. Stability ball hip extension hold		10 sec hold for 5 reps each side. For stenosis, keep a posterior tilt of the pelvis, focus on a small range of motion, and do not arch the back.	Page 90
8. Tube press-out		2 sets of 12 reps each side	Page 93

Table 9.6   Month 6 Exercises

9. Tube circle		2 sets of 8 reps each side in both directions	Page 94
10. Tube walk-out		2 sets of 8 reps each side (3 steps out and 3 steps back)	Page 95
11. Clock step		2 sets of 4 reps each side (12, 2, & 3 o'clock; then 12, 10, & 9 o'clock)	Page 98
12. Stand-up–sit-down		2 sets of 40 reps. For spondylolisthesis, be sure to land gently.	Page 99
13. Kneeling hip flexor stretch		30 sec hold for 2 reps each side. For spondylolisthesis, perform with a posterior tilt; do not arch the back.	Page 111
14. Strap hamstring stretch		60 sec hold for 2 reps each side	Page 113

Continuing Your Training

By the end of the sixth month, you should be able to include general weight training in your exercise program. For those with spondylolisthesis, it is important to keep the slight posterior tilt in your hips so that the back is in a safe position as you perform each exercise. The trick is to not ask too much of your body too quickly, so start small with light resistance and work your way up. I highly recommend the use of machines in this phase of training because they are a relatively safe way to get back into lifting weights. First, the seated position in which you are positioned in most machines encourages you to keep your flexion bias. Also, machines put you in a dedicated path of motion, which eliminates some of the inherent instability of free weights. This will make it easier in the beginning to focus on the exercise at hand and not on stabilizing the whole body. This may go against what some trainers have told you in the past, but you are now reintroducing your body to weight training and if you ask too much of your body, it may fail and send you backward. Keep in mind that this is temporary and you can reintroduce free weights to your routine as you get stronger. This will challenge you to stabilize in many different planes of motion and will be an important part of strength building once you're ready.

I realize, too, that not everyone belongs to a gym. In that case, you can continue to do month 5 and month 6 exercises indefinitely. But remember that the body gets used to what it does regularly and will stagnate and weaken over time if you don't change things up a bit. You can always increase reps, sets, or even hold times to jazz it up a bit. To challenge your body, I suggest the following for month 7 and beyond:

Months 7 and 11: Do month 3 exercises

Months 8 and 12: Do month 4 exercises

Month 9: Do month 5 exercises

Month 10: Do month 6 exercises

By changing up the exercises every four weeks or so, you keep the body challenged so you don't plateau. The body seeks homeostasis, and if you keep doing the same thing over and over again, you eventually become more efficient. This results in needing less muscle to accomplish the exercises, thus you get weaker over time. To avoid this, shake things up by doing more reps or sets, or performing the exercise for a longer period of time. All of these will work. By changing your exercise program completely (by doing the past workouts), your body never gets used to the routine and continues to stay strong.

If you need further help creating a workout program, I highly suggest hiring a personal trainer or Pilates instructor to design a program that you can follow on your own. Make sure they have some experience working with someone who has had spondylolisthesis. I also highly recommend working with someone with a Pilates background. Pilates is a great way to keep your core strong and body fit.

CHAPTER 10

Stenosis

Lumbar spinal stenosis is one of the most commonly diagnosed spinal conditions in older adults,[1] and the resulting pain can range from unnoticeable to debilitating. The diagnosis of spinal stenosis is made by a physician after a thorough examination that may include one or more of the following imaging techniques: spinal X-ray, MRI, CT scan (computed tomography), CT myelogram, and bone scan. There is some debate as to whether there has been a recent increase in the number of spinal stenosis cases. Or are there simply more cases being diagnosed because we now have better tools at our disposal for diagnosing? Stenosis is also one of the most common reasons for spinal surgery.[2,3] However, stenosis doesn't necessarily have to be a debilitating condition. In fact, one study reported that as many as 50 percent of those studied over the age of 40 were asymptomatic (no symptoms of lower back pain) yet under imaging had a diagnosis of stenosis.[4] Stenosis is a manageable condition and patients can often live relatively pain-free with proper treatment and follow-up exercise.

Definition

While there are two forms of stenosis, primary and secondary or degenerative, we will be talking mostly about secondary or degenerative spinal stenosis. Primary spinal stenosis refers to stenosis that occurs due to a congenital abnormality or a disorder of postnatal development, and it is present at a much younger age.[5] Secondary or degenerative spinal stenosis is the narrowing of either the central spinal canal or the intervertebral foramen of the spine. This narrowing can be the result of a decrease of disc height, a bulging or herniated disc, hypertrophy (increased size) of the ligamentum flavum (spinal ligament) or facet joints, or even the formation of osteophytes (bone spurs).[6] All of these conditions can cause a narrowing of the central canal, where the spinal cord travels, or the intervertebral foramen, where the nerve roots exit the spine. These narrowing conditions cause either an impingement (squeezing) of the spinal cord or nerve root which can lead to numbness, tingling, or radiating pain through the butt, hip, or leg (on one side or both sides), or localized lower back pain. Spinal stenosis predominantly occurs in the lower three lumbar levels,[7] with the lowest level (L5-S1) being the most common because the intervertebral foramen exiting the spine are smaller at that last level.[8]

Spinal stenosis is often divided into two categories—central or lateral stenosis—depending on the location of the impingement. Central stenosis refers to the narrowing of the central canal and resulting impingement of the spinal cord. The canal is often narrowed anterior to posterior (front to back), leading to a compression of the spinal cord and restricting blood supply to the cord itself (see figure 10.1).[9] Because central stenosis affects the spinal cord, we often see symptoms manifest bilaterally (on both sides or down both legs). Lateral stenosis is the impingement of the nerve root as it branches off the spinal cord and travels through the intervertebral foramen to exit the spine (see figure 10.2). This impingement can be caused by a disc bulge or herniation, osteophyte formation, hypertrophy of the ligaments or facet joints, or a slippage of one vertebra off another (spondylolisthesis). Lateral stenosis can be felt unilaterally down one leg or bilaterally down both legs, depending on how it is impinged.

Here is a great analogy that really helps to visualize stenosis. Imagine you are driving your car down the street and you hit something head-on. The airbag inflates and pushes you back against your seat, squishing you in between the seat and airbag. In a simplistic way, this illustrates spinal stenosis. In this analogy, imagine that your body is the spinal cord and your outstretched arms are the nerve roots. You are being impinged by the airbag. If the airbag is impinging you at your shoulder and arm on one side then it would be lateral stenosis; if you are being squeezed centrally with the airbag against your body, then that would be central stenosis. The only way to decompress the nerve (you) is to move the seat or the airbag. That is often done through a change in posture or positioning, or, in serious cases, through surgery.

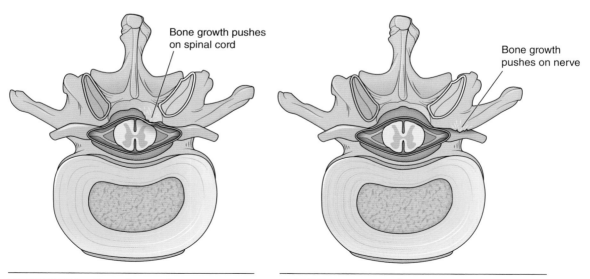

FIGURE 10.1   Central stenosis.   FIGURE 10.2   Lateral stenosis.

Symptoms

The primary symptom of stenosis is referred to as neurogenic claudication (also called pseudoclaudication). This technical term encompasses a combination of leg symptoms that affect one or more of the following: the buttocks, groin, front of the thigh, and the back side of the leg to the feet. In addition to pain, other leg symptoms can include fatigue, heaviness, weakness, and paresthesia (the tingling feeling we sometimes call "pins and needles").[6] This can be exacerbated by prolonged standing or walking. A common occurrence with stenosis, especially central stenosis, is that after walking for a particular distance, patients develop pain and discomfort down the legs. Sitting for a few moments seems to relieve the pain and discomfort because the lower spine is in a flexed position which decompresses the back enough to provide relief, and they are able to continue to walk.

Posture seems to have a direct effect on the severity of symptoms in stenosis.[10] When standing straight with "good" posture, the spine is in an extended position, which often exacerbates the narrowing of the spinal canal or intervertebral space. Individuals with stenosis usually prefer a flexed posture. This flexed posture opens up the spinal column and the space between the discs allowing a decompressing of the spinal column and nerve roots. You've probably seen this and didn't even realize it. Have you ever noticed that some older people walk with a wide gait, tailbone slung under, and a significant rounding of the low back? They probably have some stenosis. This is a posture they've adopted over time to compensate for the pain. Most people don't even realize they are doing it. Much like spondylolisthesis, the pelvis needs to be in a flexion bias during exercise, meaning that the pelvic "bowl" needs to be tipped so that if it were holding water, the water would spill out the back of the bowl (see figure 10.3). Or if you are lying down, you would flatten your back by tucking your pelvis. Flattening the spine opens up those spinal joints and decompresses the nerves. In time you may be able to get closer to a traditional neutral spine but for now it is safest to exercise with a posterior tilt in your pelvis and your back flat to the ground.

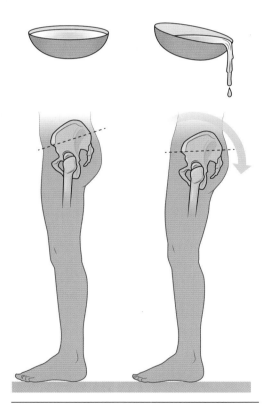

FIGURE 10.3   Visualizing the pelvis as a bowl of water in which the water spills to the back in a posterior pelvic tilt.

Contraindications

Extension of the spine is the primary contraindication. This causes a narrowing or closing of the spinal joints and often leads to increased pain, discomfort, and symptoms down the leg(s). Exercises that put the body into extension should be avoided at all cost, but any exercise that causes additional pain should be avoided. My rule of three is to perform three repetitions of the exercise to see if the pain is worse than before you started. Sometimes just the act of moving may cause some discomfort. So, if it hurts a bit on the first repetition, continue, but reevaluate after the third repetition. If the pain remains steady or increases, then stop doing that exercise for the day. Remember not every exercise is meant for everybody. Sometimes your body needs to become stronger in order to complete an exercise, so go on to the next exercise and return to the challenging one in a week or so. There's also a period of simply getting used to doing exercises in general. Once your body becomes more comfortable with doing exercise, you may find you are able to do more exercises and more repetitions.

Treatment Options

There are a variety of available treatment options for spinal stenosis depending on the severity of the condition or your symptoms. The options range from conservative to invasive. Conservative treatments are typically utilized before surgery is contemplated. Conservative treatments may include physical therapy (manual manipulation and exercise), orthotics, NSAIDs, analgesics, ice, heat, ultrasound, epidural injections, and transcutaneous electrical nerve stimulation.[6]

Spinal surgery should only be considered as a last resort when all other forms of treatment have been exhausted. The most common surgical procedure for stenosis in the last 10 years is a laminectomy, in which the nerve is decompressed by either removing the cause of the impingement, which increases the size of the intervertebral foramen, or by removing a large section of the posterior portion of the vertebrae, the lamina. Think back to the airbag analogy. A laminectomy removes the seat from behind you. The airbag is still pushing from the front but there is no impediment pushing you into the airbag from behind. By removing a portion of the vertebrae, surgeons decompress the spinal cord or nerve root. But there is a catch. When removing the lamina, doctors often remove other portions of the vertebrae, such as the spinous process or transverse process, which is determined during surgery. Remember the anatomy discussion in chapter 1? What muscles attach to the transverse and spinous processes? All of those spinal stabilizers. So, by removing a portion of the vertebrae, the spinal segments in the immediate area may become very unstable.

Another popular surgical option is spinal fusion. This is very invasive and will forever limit your spine's function. Instead of the spinal stabilizers working to stabilize the spine, post-fusion patients have two vertebrae that are fused together. Those two vertebrae are very stable and initially, the fusion may relieve the pain. However, the joint above and below the fused area will have additional stresses placed on them and can become damaged due to this increased stress.

Surgery should only be considered after nonsurgical options have been exhausted with no improvement in condition; surgery is a permanent change to your structure and should not be taken lightly. There are often resultant secondary issues that need to be weighed heavily before jumping into surgery.

Training Focus

The following exercise programs described in tables 10.1 through 10.6 will help to manage stenosis. Each month, you will either add new exercises or replace some of the current exercises with more advanced ones. The goal is progression. You want to move forward, and the only way to do that is to work a little harder by adjusting one of the variables. Those variables are volume (the number of sets and repetitions, or total number of exercises), load (the amount of weight being lifted), and frequency (the number of exercise days per week). Each month, you can look forward to a change to your routine, and as long as you are not experiencing any increased pain, you will continue with the new routine until the next month. If you have increased pain, go back to the previous month for another week or two, then give the new routine another try.

Keep in mind that not all exercises are meant for everybody. There may be an exercise that works for one person but may cause another person significant discomfort. Simply avoid any exercise that hurts. Come back to that exercise later in the month or even the following month to see if you have become strong enough to do it without pain. From my personal and professional experience, I know that there may be an exercise that you will never be able to do, and that's okay. If you cannot perform this one exercise, it will not make or break your success. Do the exercises that don't cause you pain and avoid the ones that do.

Let's discuss what kind of pain is okay and what kind is not. Normally we instruct our clients that a little discomfort is all right. On a scale of 1 to 10, with 1 being no pain at all and a 10 being the worst pain you can imagine, where would you rank your pain as you perform an exercise? If it is at a 1 to a 3, it is okay to work through it. This would include some mild discomfort. However, if the pain is severe, don't perform the exercise that day. You may feel some pain with the first or second repetition of an exercise, and want to immediately stop. I encourage you to do a couple more repetitions and see if the pain dissipates. It often will. However, if the pain continues above level 3, don't push through. Let it go for the day, and move on to the next exercise. If every exercise is causing you discomfort above a level 3, then lay off the exercises for a day or two. Let things calm down before trying them again. If the pain persists, contact your physician.

You will begin by getting comfortable with the exercises and establishing the habit of doing them regularly. I often tell my clients to do the exercises every day. It sounds like a lot but let's face reality: Most people will do the exercises three to four times per week. That's perfect. However, when I tell them to do them three to four times per week, they may actually do it only once or twice. Success hinges on your consistency. The more you do the exercises, the stronger you will get.

For the first few exercises, I suggest using a Togu Pilates balance ball in a 12 inch (30 cm) size, which can be purchased through various online retailers including Pilates.com. I particularly like this ball because it has great tactile feedback; it is strong enough to lie on but still has some springiness to it. Regular beach balls are also a possibility; if that's what you use, I recommend a 20-inch size for most people. The beach ball is an economical option, however it won't provide the same tactile feedback as the Togu ball. Also, we will be using the Togu ball mostly deflated, about 20 to 25 percent full. I put in two big breaths when I am inflating it. Start there and see how it feels. If it feels too big, like you are too high up in the air, let some air out. You know you need more air in it if the ball bottoms out when you get on it.

Lie down with the Togu ball under your pelvis, not your low back. It should be under your sacrum, and your sacrum should be level. To find this position, I recommend laying down with the ball under your back, sitting up, and then wedging the ball under your rear end as far as you can. Once you do this, slowly curl your body down onto your back with your feet remaining on the floor and knees at approximately 90 degrees. You will know it is too high (toward your low back) if you feel as though the ball is trying to arch your back. Likewise, it is too low if it places you into a tucked position. Between the two, being slightly too low is preferable to being slightly too high, especially with stenosis.

Before You Begin: Finding Neutral Spine and Engaging Kegels

Neutral spine was first discussed in detail back in chapter 1, but it is worth repeating because it applies specifically to spinal stenosis and the exercises prescribed in the following program. When talking about low back pain, neutral spine is the spinal position you can maintain with little to no pain. The exercises should be performed in a pain-free neutral spine.

The clinical definition of *neutral spine* is the position in which the anterior superior iliac spine is on the same plane as the posterior superior iliac spine. While those anatomical landmarks mean something to many health care professionals, they don't translate nearly as well to the general population. For the rest of us, neutral spine is the position of the spine that has the least amount of stress on it, where the curves of the cervical, thoracic, and lumbar regions support each other and are able to cushion the spine optimally. We will focus primarily on the lumbar spine, but remember that if you change the angle of one region, the others will also change, for better or worse. With spinal stenosis, the pelvis should be in a flexion bias, meaning it needs to be in a posterior tilt throughout all the exercises. This position will be considered your neutral spine. This flexed spinal posture will open up the spinal segments and help to decompress the nerves. The amount of flex will vary from person to person.

You will see that the first exercise in month 1 is to find your neutral spine and maintain it. Lie down (supine) on your back in a position that produces little to no pain, or such that the pain subsides as you continue to relax on your back. Next, find your Kegel muscles. These are usually described as the muscles that help to hold back a stream of urine. They are your pelvic floor muscles, a muscle group that comprises part of your inner core, and they should be slightly engaged during these exercises. Don't grip them hard, just a light hold: think 30 percent of your maximum. Hold for about 20 to 30 seconds. As you become stronger, it will become easier to maintain. Focus on keeping the muscles engaged throughout each exercise. It may not be easy, and you may forget. Once you can find neutral spine and engage the pelvic floor muscles, it's time to move on to the exercises.

Table 10.1   Month 1 Exercises

1. Neutral spine and Kegel		Hold for 30 sec	
2. Togu pelvic tilt (with hold)		5 reps of 5 sec hold for 2 sets	Page 65
3. Togu pelvic tilt		2 sets of 10 reps	Page 65
4. Togu marching		2 sets of 10 reps each side (alternating)	Page 66
5. Lying lumbar stretch		30 sec hold for 2 reps	Page 114
6. Heel slide		2 sets of 10 reps each side. For stenosis, perform with a flattened back; do not let the back arch as you extend the leg.	Page 56
7. Bent-knee fallout		2 sets of 10 reps each side. For stenosis, perform with a flattened back.	Page 55
8. Cat and cow		2 sets of 12 reps. For stenosis, focus only on the rounding of the back; do not arch the back.	Page 103

Table 10.1   Month 1 Exercises

9. Doorway hamstring stretch		60 sec hold for 2 reps. For ste-nosis, keep the opposite knee bent and the back flat.	Page 112
10. Knee-to-chest stretch		30 sec hold for 2 reps each side	Page 116

Table 10.2   Month 2 Exercises

1. Togu pelvic tilt		2 sets of 20 reps	Page 65
2. Togu marching		2 sets of 20 reps each side (alternating)	Page 66
3. Togu tilted march-up		2 sets of 8 reps each side (alternating)	Page 67
4. Togu leg lowering with pelvic tilt		2 sets of 8 reps each side (alternating)	Page 68
5. Lying lumbar stretch		30 sec hold for 2 reps	Page 114

(Continued)

Table 10.2 Month 2 Exercises *(continued)*

6. Heel slide		2 sets of 20 reps each side	Page 56
7. Lying overhead reach		2 sets of 10 reps each side	Page 63
8. Dying bug		2 sets of 8 reps each side	Page 61
9. Quadruped hold with opposite-arm tap		2 sets of 12 reps each side	Page 77
10. Quadruped hip extension slide		2 sets of 10 reps each side	Page 78
11. Strap hamstring stretch		60 sec hold for 2 reps each side	Page 113
12. Knee-to-chest stretch		30 sec hold for 2 reps each side	Page 116

Table 10.3   Month 3 Exercises

1. Togu pelvic tilt		2 sets of 20 reps.	Page 65
2. Togu tilted march-up		2 sets of 8 reps each side (alternating)	Page 67
3. Togu leg lowering with pelvic tilt		2 sets of 8 reps each side (alternating)	Page 68
4. Lying lumbar stretch		30 sec hold for 2 reps	Page 114
5. Dying bug		2 sets of 12 reps each side. For stenosis, perform with a flat back.	Page 61
6. Articulating bridge		2 sets of 12 reps. For stenosis, focus on the pelvic tilt.	Page 108
7. Pelvic press hold		5 sec hold for 5 reps. For stenosis, place a pillow under the stomach and allow a posterior tilt of the pelvis.	Page 70
8. Pelvic press hip extension		2 sets of 8 reps each side. For stenosis, place a pillow under the stomach, allow a posterior tilt of the pelvis, and focus on a small range of motion.	Page 71

(Continued)

Table 10.3   Month 3 Exercises *(continued)*

9. Quadruped hold with opposite-arm tap		2 sets of 12 reps each side	Page 77
10. Quadruped hip extension slide		2 sets of 8 reps each side. For stenosis, keep slightly tucked under through-out; do not arch the back.	Page 78
11. Quadruped hip extension lift		2 sets of 8 reps each side. For stenosis, keep slightly tucked under through-out; do not arch the back.	Page 79
12. Kneeling hip flexor stretch		30 sec hold for 2 reps each side. For steno-sis, perform with a posterior tilt; do not arch the back.	Page 111
13. Strap hamstring stretch		60 sec hold for 2 reps each side	Page 113

Table 10.4 Month 4 Exercises

1. Togu pelvic tilt		2 sets of 20 reps	Page 65
2. Togu tilted march-up		2 sets of 8 reps each side (alternating)	Page 67
3. Togu leg lowering with pelvic tilt		2 sets of 8 reps each side (alternating)	Page 68
4. Lying lumbar stretch		30 sec hold for 2 reps	Page 114
5. Dying bug		2 sets of 12 reps each side. For stenosis, perform with a flat back.	Page 61
6. Articulating bridge		2 sets of 12 reps. For stenosis, focus on the pelvic tilt.	Page 108
7. Pelvic press hip extension		2 sets of 8 reps each side. For stenosis, place a pillow under the stomach, allow a posterior tilt of the pelvis, and focus on a small range of motion.	Page 71

(Continued)

Table 10.4   Month 4 Exercises *(continued)*

8. Pelvic press shoulder retraction		5 reps of 1 sec hold. For stenosis, place a pillow under the stomach and allow a posterior tilt of the pelvis.	Page 72
9. Stability ball seated knee lift		2 sets of 8 reps each side	Page 88
10. Stability ball walk-out		2 sets of 8 reps. Begin walk-out with posterior tilt.	Page 89
11. Stability ball hip extension hold		5 reps of 5 sec hold for 2 sets each side. For stenosis, keep a posterior tilt of the pelvis, focus on a small range of motion, and do not arch the back.	Page 90
12. Stand-up–sit-down		2 sets of 25 reps. For stenosis, be sure to land gently.	Page 99

Table 10.4 Month 4 Exercises

13. Kneeling hip flexor stretch		30 sec hold for 2 reps each side. For stenosis, perform with a posterior tilt of the pelvis; do not arch the back.	Page 111
14. Strap hamstring stretch		60 sec hold for 2 reps each side	Page 113

Table 10.5 Month 5 Exercises

1. Togu pelvic tilt		2 sets of 20 reps	Page 65
2. Togu tilted march-up		2 sets of 8 reps each side (alternating)	Page 67
3. Togu tilted leg lowering		2 sets of 8 reps each side (alternating)	Page 68
4. Lying lumbar stretch		30 sec hold for 2 reps	Page 114
5. Articulating bridge		2 sets of 12 reps. For stenosis, focus on the pelvic tilt.	Page 108

(Continued)

Table 10.5   Month 5 Exercises *(continued)*

6. Full plank		3 reps of 10 sec hold for 2 sets with 3 sec rest between reps	Page 82
7. Stability ball walk-out		2 sets of 8 reps. Begin walk-out with posterior tilt.	Page 89
8. Stability ball hip extension hold		5 reps of 10 sec hold for 2 sets each side. For stenosis, keep a posterior tilt of the pelvis, focus on a small range of motion, and do not arch the back.	Page 90
9. Tube press-out		2 sets of 12 reps each side	Page 93
10. Tube circle		2 sets of 8 reps each side in both directions	Page 94

Table 10.5   Month 5 Exercises

11. Clock step		2 sets of 4 reps each side (12, 2, & 3 o'clock; then 12, 10, & 9 o'clock)	Page 98
12. Stand-up–sit-down		2 sets of 40 reps. For stenosis, be sure to land gently.	Page 99
13. Kneeling hip flexor stretch		30 sec hold for 2 reps each side. For stenosis, perform with a posterior tilt of the pelvis; do not arch the back.	Page 111
14. Strap hamstring stretch		60 sec hold for 2 reps each side	Page 113

Table 10.6 Month 6 Exercises

1. Togu pelvic tilt		2 sets of 20 reps	Page 65
2. Togu tilted march-up		2 sets of 8 each side (alternating)	Page 67
3. Togu leg lowering with pelvic tilt		2 sets of 8 reps each side (alternating)	Page 68
4. Lying lumbar stretch		30 sec hold for 2 reps	Page 114
5. Articulating bridge		2 sets of 12 reps. For stenosis, focus on the pelvic tilt.	Page 108
6. Full plank		3 reps of 10 sec hold for 2 sets with 3 sec rest between reps	Page 82
7. Stability ball hip extension hold		5 reps of 10 sec hold each side. For stenosis, keep a posterior tilt of the pelvis, focus on a small range of motion, and do not arch the back.	Page 90
8. Tube walk-out		2 sets of 8 reps each side (3 steps out and 3 steps back)	Page 95
9. Tube single-arm row		2 sets of 12 reps each side	Page 96

Table 10.6 Month 6 Exercises

10. Tube single-arm press		2 sets of 12 reps each side	Page 97
11. Clock step		2 sets of 4 reps each side (12, 2, & 3 o'clock; then 12, 10, & 9 o'clock)	Page 98
12. Stand-up–sit-down		2 sets of 50 reps. For stenosis, be sure to land gently.	Page 99
13. Step-up		2 sets of 15 reps each side on standard step (8 inches high)	Page 100
14. Kneeling hip flexor stretch		30 sec hold for 2 reps each side. For stenosis, perform with a posterior tilt of the pelvis; do not arch the back.	Page 111
15. Strap hamstring stretch		60 sec hold for 2 reps each side	Page 113

Continuing Your Training

By the end of the sixth month, you should be able to add general fitness activities to your exercise routine. An important focus for those with stenosis is to always be mindful of posture. Over time you may notice that you don't need to stay in a pronounced posterior tilt, or that your posterior tilt has slightly relaxed and you are able to exercise in a more neutral spine without pain. This is a good thing, but please be mindful that the safest position for you will be slightly tucked under, allowing for the spinal foramen to open a bit.

If you are returning to the gym, I recommend the use of machines, especially if you need to be in a posterior tilt. Most machines place you in a seated position which promotes a flexed posture, so these exercises may be a bit safer for those with stenosis. They also keep you in a dedicated path of motion which eliminates some of the inherent instability of free weights. That said, like any weightlifting activity, you need to be realistic about your abilities and goals. As you become more comfortable with lifting, feel free to utilize the free weights—in the end they will give you more bang for your buck by forcing you to stabilize the weight by using more joints.

I realize, too, that not everyone belongs to a gym. In that case, you can continue to do month 5 and month 6 exercises indefinitely. But remember that the body gets used to what it does regularly and will stagnate and weaken over time if you don't change things up a bit. To challenge your body, I suggest the following for month 7 and beyond:

Months 7 and 11: Do month 3 exercises

Months 8 and 12: Do month 4 exercises

Month 9: Do month 5 exercises

Month 10: Do month 6 exercises

By changing up the exercises every four weeks or so, you keep the body challenged so you don't plateau. The body seeks homeostasis, and if you keep doing the same thing over and over again, you eventually become more efficient. This results in needing less muscle to accomplish the exercises, and so you get weaker over time. To avoid this, shake things up by doing more reps or sets, or performing the exercise for a longer period of time. All of these will work. By changing your exercise program completely (by doing the past workouts), your body never gets used to the routine and continues to stay strong.

If you need further help creating a workout program, I highly suggest hiring a personal trainer or Pilates instructor to design a program that you can follow on your own. Make sure they have some experience working with someone who has had stenosis. I also highly recommend working with someone with a Pilates background. Pilates is a great way to keep your core strong and body fit.

CHAPTER 11

Spinal Surgeries

If you're reading this chapter, I'm assuming that by this point you've tried everything to rid yourself of your low back pain—medications for the inflammation, physical therapy to strengthen the muscles, epidural shots to calm down the nerves—and none of these have worked. It's only after exhausting all other options that you and your physician should consider surgery. And even then, there may be other surgical options to consider before choosing spinal fusion, which should be considered the last resort in spinal surgery.

Nonsurgical Options Before Surgery

A doctor's first course of action is usually to reduce the inflammation, which is why anti-inflammatories are often the first line of treatment. One theory, the Law of Pain, argues that all pain is caused by some type of inflammation, and that there are different inflammatory biochemical reactions that occur in the body depending on the condition. Arthritis, fibromyalgia, low back pain, and other conditions all have a different "inflammatory soup" of biochemical reactions that lead to pain.[1] So not all pain is the same, but it is often inflammation that leads to pain.

The doctor will first try to soothe the area and reduce the inflammation as noninvasively as possible. Rest, ice, and medications are often chosen first, with nonsteroidal anti-inflammatory drugs (NSAIDs), acetaminophen, muscle relaxants, and steroids being the most common medications prescribed. The next step is typically physical therapy, which is also noninvasive and may be used in conjunction with medication. Physical therapy can be extremely valuable, but much like a surgeon, the talent and experience of the physical therapist has a lot to do with your success. Seek out the best you can find; it's worth the effort.

Only when those options have been exhausted should the doctor take the next step and consider a minimally invasive route, such as an epidural steroid injection or nerve blocks. Then, if unsuccessful, the question of surgery will arise. This will typically be a discectomy, laminectomy, a combination of the two, or ultimately spinal fusion. The doctor will discuss the surgical options depending on the severity of the condition.[2]

Surgical Options

All too often I see people so afraid of pain that they are willing to jump into surgery far too quickly. I've been there, and believe me, I understand. When you can't move without pain or spasm, or when the numbness and tingling won't ease up and you aren't able to get comfortable no matter what position you try, forget about sleeping comfortably—that isn't happening. Trust me, if offered what seemed to be a quick-fix surgery to take that pain away, I just might take it too. "You mean, I lie down and go to sleep and when I wake up all the nerve pain will be gone? Sign me up." What nobody tells you is that the trauma of the surgery will leave you with a different pain than your original discomfort. The recovery isn't easy. In fact, depending on the surgery, you need to be prepared for up to six to twelve months of therapy and continual post-surgery exercise. People have come to me years after surgery saying they still have some pain on a daily basis. The pain is not the same as before the surgery, but there is still pain and discomfort. To some degree, this is the client's responsibility: If a person doesn't keep up their physical therapy exercises, the back becomes unstable and the pain returns.

The most common symptom that raises the surgery question is radiculopathy. Radiating pain, numbness, and tingling down the leg can eventually develop into a great enough nerve disruption that you acquire motor function disorder and weakness in your leg (such as drop foot) or a serious condition called cauda equina syndrome (see sidebar on page 203). Let me explain how an impingement of the nerves in the spine could cause radiculopathy. Imagine you are driving your car down the street and you hit something head-on. The airbag inflates and pushes you back against your seat, squishing you in between the seat and airbag. In a simplistic way, that is what is happening in your spine. In this analogy, imagine that your body is the spinal cord and your outstretched arms are the nerve roots. You (the spinal cord and nerves) are being impinged by the airbag (which represents the nucleus pulposus of the disc protruding out and into the foramen) and the seat behind (the bones of the vertebrae itself). The only way to decompress the nerve (you) is to move either the seat or the airbag. A discectomy is removal of the airbag, or a portion of it, and a laminectomy is the removal of the seat, which we discuss later in this section.

Each surgery option has benefits and drawbacks. The more knowledge you have about them, the better choices you can make for your health. And when it comes to spinal surgery, these choices may affect the rest of your life, so make sure you know before you go.

The most popular surgery for solving disc issues, like a disc herniation with radiculopathy, is a discectomy.[4] The traditional method is referred to as an open discectomy. This is a more invasive technique in which an incision is made to remove a portion of the disc that affects the nerve root (see figure 11.1), and may be used in conjunction with a laminectomy, explained later in this section. The outcomes for open discectomy are considered good to excellent.

The second type of discectomy, and one that is becoming increasingly popular, is the less invasive microdiscectomy, which is usually done arthroscopically. This surgery's goal is nearly identical to the open discectomy; the primary difference is that the microdiscectomy is done with imaging technology, such

What is Cauda Equina Syndrome?

There are times when immediate spinal surgery is the only option. The back pain may be the result of something called cauda equina syndrome (CES), defined by the American Association of Neurological Surgeons as a condition that occurs when the nerve roots of the cauda equina (nerves at the end of the spinal cord) are compressed enough to disrupt motor and sensory function to the lower extremities and bladder. This is a medical emergency and surgery is necessary. Usually caused by a massively herniated disc, CES is associated with low back pain and will often be accompanied by red-flag symptoms,[3] such as:

- Severe low back pain
- Motor weakness, sensory loss, or pain in one or both legs
- Bladder or bowel dysfunction and incontinence
- Sexual dysfunction
- A loss of reflexes in the lower extremities

This condition occurs in a very small percentage of people with low back pain and is diagnosed by a physician. It often requires immediate surgery. If at any time you exhibit any of the symptom of CES, seek medical attention as soon as possible.

as a special microscope, which makes a smaller incision and protects the soft tissues and muscles as much as possible. This technique offers less soft tissue damage, blood loss, operating time, hospital stay, and a quicker recovery.[5] The primary difference between the two methods involves the skill of the surgeon. The microdiscectomy has a steeper learning curve and requires greater technical skill in the use of specialized equipment and navigation systems to accomplish the surgery.

Another common surgical procedure is a laminectomy with discectomy. Surgeons are able to first decompress the nerve by either increasing the size of the intervertebral foramen or removing a large section of the posterior portion of the vertebrae (the lamina), and then remove a chunk of the nucleus pul-

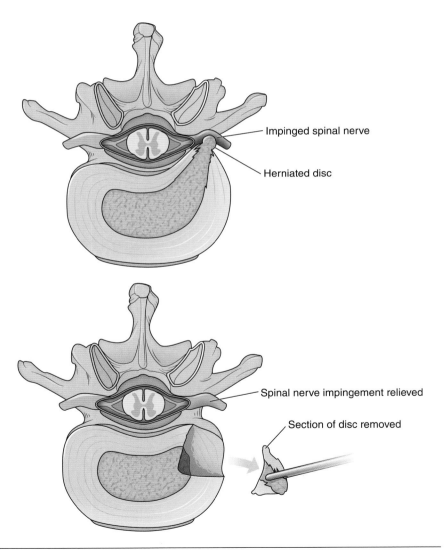

FIGURE 11.1   Open discectomy.

posus that is pinching off the nerve (see figure 11.2). Remember the analogy about the airbag? The airbag is the herniated disc, you are the nerve and nerve roots, and the seat is the bony structures of the vertebra. In this analogy, the laminectomy removes the seat from behind you. The airbag is still pushing from the front, but now there is no impediment pushing you forward into the airbag from behind. By removing a portion of the vertebrae, the spinal cord or nerve root is decompressed. But there is a catch. When removing the lamina, doctors often determine that they also need to remove other portions of the vertebrae, such as the spinous processes or transverse processes. Remember the anatomy section that described the spinal stabilizers and how they attach to the transverse and spinous processes? By removing a portion of the verte-

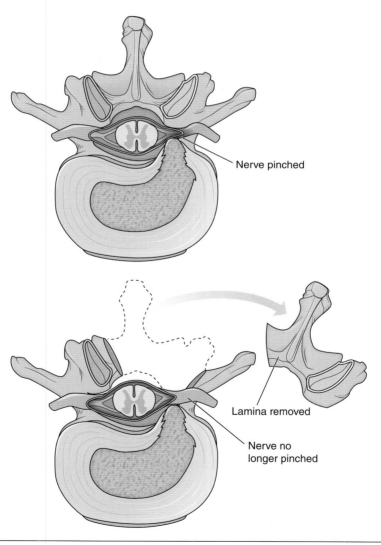

FIGURE 11.2   Laminectomy, or removal of the lamina to decompress a nerve.

brae, the spinal segments in the immediate area may become very unstable. And since the vertebrae are removed, there is an inherently weak and unstable portion of your spine. Other lumbar muscles will need to assume the job of stabilizing of the spine to keep it stable and strong.

Statistically, there are no differences between the outcomes of these two types of surgeries. Good or excellent results average at 79 percent, with the best long-term results (85%) coming from the microdiscectomy. Much of the success of either type of surgery depends on the skill of the surgeon and the client's post-surgery rehabilitation.[13]

The next, and typically final step, is spinal fusion surgery. It is usually the last choice because it is permanent and there is no going back afterward, so it should only be considered after all other options are exhausted.

Spinal fusion surgeries are still considered the gold standard for certain spinal conditions, and more people are having them each year. In 1998, there were 174,223 spinal fusion surgeries. Compare that to 2008, in which there were 413,174 surgeries, with the greatest increase being in the lumbar region, an increase of 142 percent.[6]

The process of spinal fusion surgery is actually simple in nature. The physician essentially removes the disc and fuses one vertebrae to the adjacent vertebrae. There are a few different methods that can also be combined with one another. The surgeon makes the decision based on the specific case and condition.

The first method uses an interbody spacer. This is a device made out of titanium, either solid in construction or hollow (to be filled with a bone graft) that takes the place of the disc. It is approximately the same height as the disc and is placed between the bodies of the vertebrae after the disc has been removed. This decompresses the nerves by increasing the space in the intervertebral foramen allowing more room for the nerves. If there is a bone graft placed within the cage appliance, this bone graft will then grow and ultimately fuse the bones together.[7]

A second method attaches rods or plates to the posterior aspect of the vertebrae with pedicle screws. For a single fusion (one vertebra to another), plates or rods are used to fixate the vertebrae together. For multilevel fusions, rods are often used because they can be arranged individually and shaped as necessary. They are attached posteriorly on the vertebrae between the spinous and transverse processes (the pedicle) with pedicle screws, and the rods or plates lock the vertebrae in place. There are occasions, though rare, that some of the spinal stabilizer muscles are kept intact, although they are often removed during the surgery.[7]

Two common incision approaches to the surgery are anterior (through the stomach) and posterior (through the back). The posterior approach is used when posterior decompression is needed, when the space in the back of the vertebrae needs to be increased to take pressure off the nerves. This approach would be used for severe stenosis or if the intervertebral foramen has been occluded by bone spurs, hypertrophied facet joints, or degenerative disc disease. The anterior approach is used when the pain is primarily caused by the disc and a posterior decompression isn't necessary.[9] The advantages are that the posterior muscles aren't disturbed and the spinal stabilizers are kept intact. The approach used ultimately depends on the specific case and condition of the patient, as well as the physician's preference.

It can take six to twelve months to recover from spinal fusion surgery before you will feel close to 100 percent, although many factors go into this, including age, fitness level, and overall health. The first four to six weeks are the most difficult. Most people return to work after one to three months if their job is sedentary. Those with light-duty jobs, in which some lifting may be required, may need longer healing time before returning to work. I highly recommend working with a physical therapist after surgery, which will most likely be prescribed by your physician. In physical therapy, you may learn how to brace using your abdominals (which is discussed in the next section), how to move while protecting your spine, and how to accomplish activities of daily life. You would be surprised at how difficult everyday tasks, like tying your shoes and putting on pants, can be post-surgery. I tell everyone who has to go through a surgery that you only get to rehab properly one time, so give it all you've got and make the most of it. If you blow it off or don't take it seriously, it will come back to bite you down the road. If you don't follow the rehab instructions carefully, you may never regain full use of your body, and may have to go through the rehab process again, only this time it will be more difficult and will take a lot longer.

As with most surgeries, there are both positives and negatives to spinal fusion surgery. The best outcome is that the nerve pain is eliminated. I've had clients wake from surgery and tell me that for the first time they can remember, the nerve pain is gone. You can visibly see the relief they feel because they don't have the constant numbness, tingling, or radiating pain that they've endured for so long. Another positive is that the dysfunctional and unstable spinal joint is now incredibly stable. It's incredibly weak, but stable.

The negative facets start with the spinal structure, because it has been permanently altered. It will never be the same as it was before the surgery. Much like a car that was in a major wreck, no matter how skillful the mechanics and technicians are, that car will never be as strong and as solid as when it left the showroom floor. They can only do so much to make it as functional as possible. Another negative is that because the spinal joint is now fused, it has no motion at all. From a stability standpoint, this is great: It is a really stable joint. Unfortunately, the spine was meant to move; we are not statues. Because this spinal joint no longer moves, the joints above and below the fusion will have increased stress placed on them to accomplish the same amount of motion and flexibility the spine once allowed. This can lead to the adjacent spinal joints becoming damaged: We often see disc herniations occur at the adjacent spinal joints over time. The limited range of motion of the spine needs to be respected. People who have had spinal fusion surgery often try to increase the range of motion of their spine, but they don't realize that this type of motion is contraindicated for their condition—there is simply no spinal motion to achieve without damaging other nearby structures. Well-intentioned advice from a yoga teacher or fitness professional about the need for more flexibility can lead fusion patients down the wrong path. Spinal fusion will always create restrictions when it comes to your spinal range of motion.

Training Focus

The exercise programs described in tables 11.1 through 11.6 in this section should only be done after you have completed your post-surgical physical therapy. When you complete therapy, the therapist often gives a number of exercises for you to continue to do at home. Follow this regimen for some time. The therapist knows your body and may have customized these exercise choices specifically for your body. The exercises I include here can be used in conjunction with those provided to you from the therapist, and by those who are further down the road of recovery and need a jump-start to get back on track to see more progress. These exercises will help you to become stronger and get back to fitness, a bridge between your rehab and general fitness.

I briefly mentioned abdominal bracing when discussing physical therapy. This is a technique you will most likely learn fresh out of surgery. Many therapists utilize it post-surgery because it gets people to think about keeping their abdominals engaged whenever they move. Abdominal bracing has been demonstrated as being one of the most effective exercise techniques for abdominal stability. In fact, it has been shown to increase the stiffness of the spine, promoting stability in the individual vertebral segments[8,9] and continues to be one of the most popular abdominal strengthening techniques in rehabilitation.[10] In a nutshell, bracing is an isometric cocontraction of all the layers of the abdominals. It is the feeling of tightening your abdominals and pushing them out at the same time (similar to bearing down when having a bowel movement). This has been shown to increase strength in three of the four abdominal muscles; rectus abdominis, external oblique, and internal oblique.[11] To activate and strengthen the other abdominal muscle, the transversus abdominus, there is a technique known as abdominal hollowing. This is accomplished by drawing in your abdominals and is a great way to activate the deepest layer of the abdominals, transverse abdominus. It is superior to bracing in strengthening this deep layer.[12] If you have been taught to brace while doing your abdominal exercises, that's fine. And continue to do it if you feel it is helping. But there usually comes a time when you need to move beyond it, when you need to remember how to move properly without feeling any strain in your abdominal muscles. That's what these exercises are designed to do, to go beyond bracing and into real life.

During physical therapy, you may have been taught to flatten your back completely during exercises. This is okay too, and continue to follow that advice if it feels right for you, but I'd like to challenge you and allow you to ease up on that a bit. It is okay if your back isn't slammed flat down. Having a tiny arch to a neutral spine is natural and your back should be able to do this, as long as you don't fall into the habit of creating a big arch.

Why am I bringing this up? When people learn to brace, they are often taught to push their low back into the floor as hard as they can. Some may even be pushing into a device like a blood pressure cuff, to measure how hard they are pushing. At the beginning, this is great. However, bracing increases intra-abdominal pressure to a significant degree, which is called a Valsalva maneuver. It raises a person's blood pressure, and doing this constantly during all exercises becomes counterproductive down the road. You should not grip or strain your abdominal muscles, and flatten your back every time you exercise. There needs to come a point in which the muscles know their job and are able to fire as they were designed. That's where we are heading with the following exercises.

Positioning focuses on a neutral spine unless you have been told otherwise; in that case, follow the advice of your doctor or physical therapist. We are going to spend the first month focusing on spinal stability exercises again, which may seem familiar to you. We need to reeducate your core on how to support your body and stabilize your spine again.

Table 11.1   Month 1 Exercises

1. Bent-knee fallout		2 sets of 10 reps each side	Page 55
2. Heel slide		2 sets of 10 reps each side	Page 56
3. Marching		2 sets of 10 reps each side (alternating)	Page 57
4. March-up		2 sets of 8 reps each side (alternating)	Page 58
5. Lying overhead reach		2 sets of 12 reps each side	Page 63
6. Pelvic press hold		5 sec hold for 5 reps	Page 70
7. Pelvic press hip extension		2 sets of 10 reps each side	Page 71
8. Pelvic press shoulder retraction		5 reps of 5 sec hold for 2 sets	Page 72

Table 11.1   Month 1 Exercises

9. Quadruped hold with opposite-arm tap		8 reps of 2 sec hold each side for 2 sets	Page 77
10. Quadruped hip extension slide		2 sets of 12 reps each side	Page 78
11. Doorway hamstring stretch		30 sec hold for 2 sets each side	Page 112
12. Supine or seated piriformis stretch		30 sec hold for 2 sets each side	Page 118 or 119

Table 11.2   Month 2 Exercises

1. Bent-knee fallout		2 sets of 15 reps each side	Page 55
2. March-up		2 sets of 15 reps each side (alternating)	Page 58
3. Leg lowering		2 sets of 10 reps each side (alternating)	Page 59
4. Dying bug		2 sets of 10 reps each side	Page 61
5. Pelvic press shoulder retraction		8 reps of 5 sec hold for 2 sets	Page 72
6. Pelvic press W		5 reps of 5 sec hold for 2 sets	Page 73
7. Quadruped birddog		8 reps of 1 sec hold each side for 2 sets	Page 80
8. High plank		30 sec hold for 2 sets	Page 81
9. Side plank		10-15 sec hold for 2 reps each side. For spinal fusion, if you don't have the strength for the full version, perform on the knees.	Page 83

Table 11.2 Month 2 Exercises

10. Stability ball hip extension hold		5 reps of 5 sec hold for 2 sets each side. For stenosis, keep a posterior tilt of the pelvis, focus on a small range of motion, and do not arch the back.	Page 90
11. Kneeling hip flexor stretch		60 sec hold for 2 reps each side	Page 111
12. Doorway hamstring stretch		60 sec hold for 2 reps each side	Page 112
13. Supine or seated piriformis stretch		60 sec hold for 2 reps each side	Page 118 or 119

Table 11.3   Month 3 Exercises

1. Dying bug		2 sets of 12 reps each side	Page 61
2. Advanced kick-out		2 sets of 8 reps each side	Page 60
3. Full plank		5 reps of 10 sec hold for 2 sets with 3 sec hold between reps	Page 82
4. Side plank		10-15 sec hold for 2 reps each side. For spinal fusion, if you don't have the strength for the full version, perform on the knees.	Page 83
5. Quadruped birddog		2 sets of 15 reps each side	Page 80
6. Stability ball hip extension hold		10 reps of 5 sec hold for 2 sets each side. For stenosis, keep a posterior tilt of the pelvis, focus on a small range of motion, and do not arch the back.	Page 90
7. Tube press-out		2 sets of 12 reps each side	Page 93

Table 11.3   Month 3 Exercises

8. Tube circle		2 sets of 12 reps each side in both directions	Page 94
9. Stand-up–sit-down		2 sets of 20 reps	Page 99
10. Step-up		2 sets of 20 reps each side	Page 100
11. Kneeling hip flexor stretch		60 sec hold for 2 reps each side	Page 111
12. Strap hamstring stretch		60 sec hold for 2 reps each side	Page 113
13. Supine or seated piriformis stretch		60 sec hold for 2 reps each side	Page 118 or 119

Table 11.4   Month 4 Exercises

1. Dying bug		2 sets of 16 reps each side	Page 61
2. Advanced kick-out		2 sets of 12 reps each side	Page 60
3. Full plank		8 reps of 10 sec hold for 2 sets with 3 sec rest between reps	Page 82
4. Side plank		10-15 sec hold for 2 reps each side. For spinal fusion, if you don't have the strength for the full version, perform on the knees.	Page 83
5. Quadruped bird-dog		2 sets of 15 reps each side	Page 80
6. Ball birddog		8 reps of 2 sec hold each side for 2 sets. Stay in a posterior tilt.	Page 91
7. Tube circle		2 sets of 15 reps each side in both directions	Page 94

Table 11.4   Month 4 Exercises

8. Tube walk-out		2 sets of 15 reps each side (one step to the side)	Page 95
9. Stand-up–sit-down (single-leg)		2 sets of 8 reps each side. For spinal fusion, if single leg is too difficult, perform using both legs.	Page 99
10. Step-up		2 sets of 30 reps each side	Page 100
11. Kneeling hip flexor stretch		60 sec hold for 2 reps each side	Page 111
12. Strap hamstring stretch		60 sec hold for 2 reps each side	Page 113
13. Supine or seated piriformis stretch		60 sec hold for 2 reps each side	Page 118 or 119

Table 11.5   Month 5 Exercises

1. Dying bug		2 sets of 16 reps each side	Page 61
2. Full plank		30 sec hold for 3 reps	Page 82
3. Side plank		30 sec hold for 2 reps each side. For spinal fusion, if you don't have the strength for the full version, perform on the knees.	Page 83
4. Quadruped birddog		2 sets of 15 reps each side	Page 80
5. Ball birddog		8 reps of 2 sec hold each side for 2 sets. Stay in a posterior tilt.	Page 91
6. Pelvic press W		5 reps of 5 sec hold for 2 sets	Page 73
7. Pelvic press T		5 reps of 5 sec hold for 2 sets	Page 74
8. Tube walk-out		2 sets of 10 reps each side (2 steps to the side)	Page 95

Table 11.5   Month 5 Exercises

9. Stand-up–sit-down (single-leg)		2 sets of 15 reps each side. If single leg is too difficult continue performing with both legs.	Page 99
10. Step-up		2 sets of 30 reps each side with 5-10 lb weight in one hand	Page 100
11. Kneeling hip flexor stretch		60 sec hold for 2 reps each side	Page 111
12. Strap hamstring stretch		60 sec hold for 2 reps each side	Page 113
13. Supine or seated piriformis stretch		60 sec hold for 2 reps each side	Page 118 or 119

Table 11.6   Month 6 Exercises

1. Full plank		30 sec hold for 3 reps	Page 82
2. Side plank		30 sec hold for 2 reps each side For spinal fusion, if you don't have the strength for the full version, perform on the knees.	Page 83
3. Ball birddog		8 reps of 2 sec hold each side for 2 sets. Stay in a posterior tilt.	Page 91
4. Pelvic press W		5 reps of 5 sec hold for 2 sets	Page 73
5. Pelvic press T		5 reps of 5 sec hold for 2 sets	Page 74
6. Tube walk-out		2 sets of 10 reps each side (2 steps to the side)	Page 95
7. Tube circle		2 sets of 10 reps in each direction	Page 94
8. Stand-up–sit-down (single-leg)		2 sets of 15 reps each side. If single leg is too difficult, continue performing with both legs.	Page 99

Table 11.6   Month 6 Exercises

9. Step-up		2 sets of 30 reps each side with 5-10 lb weight in one hand	Page 100
10. Tube single-arm row		2 sets of 15 reps each side. Make sure to keep the torso still and limit rotation to the shoulders.	Page 96
11. Tube single-arm press		2 sets of 15 reps each side. Make sure to keep the torso still and limit rotation to the shoulders.	Page 97
12. Kneeling hip flexor stretch		60 sec hold for 2 reps each side	Page 111
13. Strap hamstring stretch		60 sec hold for 2 reps each side	Page 113
14. Supine or seated piriformis stretch		60 sec hold for 2 reps each side	Page 118 or 119

Continuing Your Training

By the end of the sixth month you should be able to include more general fitness activities to your exercise routine. That said, you will still need to be mindful of remaining stable throughout your core. Remember that while the fusion is very stable, the spinal joints above and below the fusion are more susceptible to injury if too much range of motion is asked of them. Keep this in mind when you are doing the exercises and avoid extreme ranges of motion. Be cautious with activities like yoga or stretch classes. Group instructors typically have the best of intentions, but they may unwittingly ask you to go beyond the capabilities of your spine. You don't want to damage another disc, so be cautious with spinal flexion, extension, and lateral flexion, and especially rotation. Remember that your lumbar spine doesn't want to rotate, so don't force it. That is a sure recipe for additional injury.

When returning to the gym, I recommend the use of machines, especially if you need to be in a posterior tilt. Most machines place you in a seated position which promotes the posterior tilt, so it will be a bit safer in general. Machines also keep you in a dedicated path of motion so you won't have to worry about stabilizing as much as you would with free weights. That said, like any weightlifting activity, you need to be realistic about your abilities and goals. As you become more comfortable with lifting, feel free to utilize the free weights; in the end, they will give you more bang for your buck by forcing you to stabilize the weight by using more joints.

I realize, too, that not everyone belongs to a gym. In that case, you can continue to do month 4 and month 5 exercises indefinitely. But remember that the body gets used to what it does regularly and will stagnate and weaken over time if you don't change things up a bit. You can increase reps, sets, or even hold times to jazz it up a bit. To challenge your body, I suggest the following:

Months 7 and 11: Do month 3 exercises

Months 8 and 12: Do month 4 exercises

Month 9: Do month 5 exercises

Month 10: Do month 6 exercises

This is a great way to keep your body off-kilter just enough to continue to see progress, and not plateau. Changing the reps, sets, and duration works, but changing the exercises themselves is an even better way to keep the workouts fresh. Consider the exercises you've learned in this chapter as your foundation, your anchor. They are exercises that you can return to again and again to reinforce your newfound stabilization and core strength that will help you reduce your LBP and result in a stronger body that is more resilient and resistant to injury.

If you need further help creating a workout program, I highly suggest hiring a personal trainer or Pilates instructor to design a program that you can follow on your own. Make sure they have some experience working with someone who has had spinal fusion. I highly recommend working with someone with a Pilates background. Pilates is a great way to keep your core strong and body fit.

References

Introduction

1. Sigmund Freud, *Beyond the Pleasure Principle*, the Standard Edition (New York: W.W. Norton & Company, 1990).

Chapter 1

1. D. Hoy et al., "The Global Burden of Low Back Pain: Estimates From the Global Burden of Disease 2010 Study," *Annals of the Rheumatic Diseases* 73, no. 6 (June 2014): 968-74, doi: 10.1136/annrheumdis-2013-204428.

2. "The Hidden Impact of Musculoskeletal Disorders on Americans," United State Bone and Joint Initiative, 2018, https://www.boneandjointburden.org/docs/BMUS%20Impact%20of%20MSK%20on%20Americans%20booklet_4th%20Edition%20%282018%29.pdf.

3. D.I. Rubin, "Epidemiology and Risk Factors for Spine Pain," *Neurologic Clinics* 25, no. 2 (May 2007): 353-71.

4. Agency for Health Care Policy and Research, "Project Briefs: Back Pain Patient Outcomes Assessment Team (BOAT)," *MEDTEP Update* 1, no. 1.

5. A. Thorstensson and H. Carlson, "Fibre Types in Human Lumbar Back Muscles," *Acta Physiologica Scandinavica* 131, no. 2 (Oct. 1987): 195-202.

6. B. Goff, "The Application of Recent Advances in Neurophysiology to Miss M. Rood's Concept of Neuromuscular Facilitation," *Physiotherapy* 58, no. 2 (Dec. 1972): 409-15

7. V. Janda, "Pain in the Locomotor System – A Broad Approach," In *Aspects of Manipulative Therapy*, eds. E. F. Glasgow et al. (New York: Churchill Livingstone, 1985), 148-51.

8. S. A. Sahrmann, *Diagnosis and Treatment of Movement Impairment Syndromes* (Maryland Heights, MO: Mosby, 2002).

Chapter 2

1. P. Page, C. Frank, and R. Lardner, *Assessment and Treatment of Muscular Imbalance* (Illinois: Human Kinetics, 2010), 49-50, 56-58.

2. "American Heart Association Recommendations for Physical Activity in Adults and Kids," American Heart Association, www.heart.org/en/healthy-living/fitness/fitness-basics/aha-recs-for-physical-activity-in-adults.

3. C. Lundby and R.A. Jacobs, "Adaptations of Skeletal Muscle Mitochondria to Exercise Training," *Experimental Physiology* 101, no. 1 (2016): 17-22.

4. V. Janda, "Pain in the Locomotor System – A Broad Approach," In *Aspects of Manipulative Therapy*, eds. E.F. Glasgow et al. (New York: Churchill Livingstone, 1985): 148-51.

5. Y.B. Sung, J.H. Lee, and Y.H. Park, "Effects of Thoracic Mobilization and Manipulation on Function and Mental State in Chronic Lower Back Pain," *Journal of Physical Therapy Science* 26, no. 11 (Nov. 2014): 1711-14, doi:10.1589/jpts.26.1711.

Chapter 3

1. "Back Health and Posture," Cleveland Clinic, https://my.clevelandclinic.org/health/articles/4485-back-health-and-posture.

2. A.D. Vigotsky, G.J. Lehman et al., "The Modified Thomas Test Is Not a Valid Measure of Hip Extension Unless Pelvic Tilt Is Controlled," *PeerJ* 4 (2016): e2325.

3. V. Akuthota and S.F. Nadler, "Core Strengthening," *Archives of Physical Medicine and Rehabilitation* 85, no. 3 (Mar. 2004): S86-S92.

Chapter 7

1. Federico Balagué et al., "Non-specific low back pain," *The Lancet* 379, no. 9814 (Feb. 2012): 482-91.

2. H.S. Picavet, J.N. Struijs, and G.P. Westert, "Utilization of Health Resources Due to Low Back Pain: Survey and Registered Data Compared," *Spine* (Phila Pa 1976) 33 (2008): 436-44.

3. L.J. Jeffries, S.F. Milanese, and K.A. Grimmer-Somers, "Epidemiology of Adolescent Spinal Pain: A Systematic Overview of the Research Literature," *Spine* (Phila Pa 1976) 32 (2007): 2630-7

4. R. Shiri et al., "The Association Between Obesity and Low Back Pain: A Meta-analysis," *American Journal of Epidemiology* 171 (2010): 135-54.

5. R. Shiri et al., "The Association Between Smoking and Low Back Pain: A Meta-analysis," *American Journal of Medicine* 123 (2010): 87 e7-35.

6. H. Heneweer, L. Vanhees, and H.S. Picavet, "Physical Activity and Low Back Pain: A U-Shaped Relation?" *Pain* 143 (2009): 21-5.

7. M. van Tulder, et al., "Chapter 3. European Guidelines for the Management of Acute Nonspecific Low Back Pain in Primary Care," *European Spine Journal* 15, suppl 2 (2006): S169-91.

8. M. Krismer, and M. van Tulder, "Strategies for Prevention and Management of Musculoskeletal Conditions. Low Back Pain (Non-specific)," *Best Practice & Research: Clinical Rheumatology* 21 (2007): 77-91.

Chapter 8

1. F. Postacchini, and G. Cinotti, "Etiopathogenesis," in Lumbar Disc Herniation, ed. F. Postacchini (New York: Spring-Verlag, 1999): 151-64.

2. M. Heliovaara, Epidemiology of Sciatica and Herniated Lumbar Intervertebral Disc (Helsinki, Finland: The Social Insurance Institution, 1988).

3. S. Friberg and C. Hirsch, "Anatomical and Clinical Studies on Lumbar Disc Degeneration," *Acta Orthopaedica Scandinavica* 19 (1949): 222-42.

4. Jo Jordan, Kika Konstantinou, and John O'Dowd, "Herniated Lumbar Disc," *BMJ Clinical Evidence* (2009): 1118.

5. M.C. Jensen et al., "Magnetic Resonance Imaging of the Lumbar Spine in People Without Back Pain," *New England Journal of Medicine* 331 (1994): 69-73

6. R.A. Deyo and J.N. Weinstein, "Low Back Pain," *New England Journal of Medicine* 344 (2001): 365-70.

7. L.A.C. Machado et al., "The McKenzie Method for Low Back Pain: A Systematic Review of the Literature With a Meta-Analysis Approach," *Spine* (Phila Pa 1776) 31, no. 9 (2006): E254-E262 (A1).

8. F.I. Namnaqani et al., "The Effectiveness of McKenzie Method Compared to Manual Therapy for Treating Chronic Low Back Pain: A Systematic Review," *Journal of Musculoskeletal and Neuronal Interactions* 19, no. 4 (Dec. 2019): 492-9.

Chapter 9

1. J. Fitzgerald and P.H. Newman, "Degenerative Spondylolisthesis," *Journal of Bone and Joint Surgery*. British Volume 58 (1976): 184-92.

2. M.L.P Ver , J.R. Dimar, and L.Y. Carreon, "Traumatic Lumbar Spondylolisthesis: A Systematic Review and Case Series," *Global Spine Journal* 9, no. 7 (Oct. 2019): 767-82, doi: 10.1177/2192568218801882, Epub 2018 Sep 27.

3. "Spondylolisthesis," Cleveland Clinic, https://my.clevelandclinic.org/health/diseases/10302-spondylolisthesis.

4. N. Evans and M. McCarthy, "Management of Symptomatic Degenerative Low-Grade Lumbar Spondylolisthesis," *EFORT Open Reviews* 3, no. 12 (Dec. 2018): 620-31.

5. S. Jacobsen et al., "Degenerative Lumbar Spondylolisthesis: An Epidemiological Perspective: The Copenhagen Osteoarthritis Study," *Spine* 32 (2007): 120-25.

6. S. Matsunaga et al., "Natural History of Degenerative Spondylolisthesis: Pathogenesis and Natural Course of the Slippage," *Spine* 15 (1990): 1204-10.

Chapter 10

1. Y.R. Rampersaud et al., "Assessment of Health-Related Quality of Life After Surgical Treatment of Focal Symptomatic Spinal Stenosis Compared with Osteoarthritis of the Hip or Knee," *Spine* 8, no. 2 (Mar.-Apr. 2008): 296-304, PubMed: 17669690.

2. M.A. Ciol et al., "An Assessment of Surgery for Spinal Stenosis: Time Trends, Geographic Variations, Complications, and Reoperations," *Journal of the American Geriatrics Society* 44, no 3 (Mar. 1996): 285-90, PubMed: 8600197.

3. R.A. Deyo et al., "United States Trends in Lumbar Fusion Surgery for Degenerative Conditions," *Spine* 30, no. 12 (Jun 2005): 1441-5. discussion 6–7, PubMed: 15959375.

4. S.W. Wiesel et al., "A Study of Computer-Assisted Tomography. I. The Incidence of Positive CAT Scans in an Asymptomatic Group of Patients," *Spine* 9 (1984): 549-51, PubMed: 6495024.

5. S.F. Ciricillo and P.R. Weinstein, "Lumbar Spinal Stenosis," *Western Journal of Medicine* 158, no. 2 (Feb. 1993):171-7, PubMed: 8434469.

6. S. Genevay and S.J. Atlas, "Lumbar Spinal Stenosis," *Best Practice and Research: Clinical Rheumatology* 24, no. 2 (2010): 253-65, doi:10.1016/j.berh.2009.11.001.

7. T. Amundsen et al., "Lumbar Spinal Stenosis. Clinical and Radiologic Features," *Spine* 20, no. 10 (May 1995): 1178-86, PubMed: 7638662.

8. L.G. Jenis and H.S. An, "Spine Update. Lumbar Foraminal Stenosis," *Spine* 25, no. 3 (2000): 389-94, PubMed: 10703115.

9. A. Raja et al., "Spinal Stenosis," [Updated 2019 Jul 13]. In StatPearls [Internet]. Treasure Island (FL): StatPearls Publishing; Jan. 2019.

10. D. Mazanec, V. Podichetty, and A. Hisa, "Lumbar Stenosis: Start with Nonsurgical Therapy," *Cleveland Clinic Journal of Medicine* 96 (2002).

Chapter 11

1. S. Omoigui, "The Biochemical Origin of Pain: The Origin of All Pain is Inflammation and the Inflammatory Response. Part 2 of 3 - Inflammatory Profile of Pain Syndromes," *Medical Hypotheses* 69, no. 6 (2007): 1169-78, doi:10.1016/j.mehy.2007.06.033.

2. C. Centeno et al., "Treatment of Lumbar Degenerative Disc Disease-Associated Radicular Pain with Culture-Expanded Autologous Mesenchymal Stem Cells: A Pilot Study on Safety and Efficacy," *Journal of Translational Medicine* 15, no. 1 (Sept. 2017): 197, doi:10.1186/s12967-017-1300-y.

3. "Cauda Equina Syndrome," American Association of Neurological Surgeons, www.aans.org/en/Patients/Neurosurgical-Conditions-and-Treatments/Cauda-Equina-Syndrome.

4. J. N. Weinstein et al., "Surgical vs Nonoperative Treatment for Lumbar Disk Herniation: The Spine Patient Outcomes Research Trial (SPORT) Observational Cohort." *Journal of the American Medical Association* 296, no. 20 (2006): 2451-59, doi:10.1001/jama.296.20.2451.

5. W. Jiang et al., "Feasibility and Efficacy of Percutaneous Lateral Lumbar Discectomy in the Treatment of Patients with Lumbar Disc Herniation: A Preliminary Experience," *Biomed Research International* (Jan. 2015): 378612, doi:10.1155/2015/378612.

6. S. Rajaee et al., "A Careful Analysis of Trends in Spinal Fusion in the United States from 1998 to 2008," Poster presented at Orthopaedic Research Society annual meeting, Long Beach, CA, Jan. 2011.

7. Elizabeth E. Rutherford et al., "Lumbar Spine Fusion and Stabilization: Hardware, Techniques, and Imaging Appearances," *RadioGraphics* 27, no. 6 (Nov. 2007), doi. org/10.1148/rg.276065205.

8. F.J. Vera-Garcia et al., "Effects of Different Levels of Torso Coactivation on Trunk Muscular and Kinematic Responses to Posteriorly Applied Sudden Loads," *Clinical Biomechanics* 21 (2006): 443-55.

9. F.J. Vera-Garcia et al., "Effects of Abdominal Stabilization Maneuvers on the Control of Spine Motion and Stability Against Sudden Trunk Perturbations," *Journal of Electromyography and Kinesiology* 17 (2007): 556-67.

10. M. Monfort-Panego et al., "Electromyographic Studies in Abdominal Exercises: A Literature Synthesis," *Journal of Manipulative and Physiological Therapeutics* 32 (2009), 232-44.

11. Sumiaki Maeo et al., "Trunk Muscle Activities During Abdominal Bracing: Comparison Among Muscles and Exercises," *Journal of Sports Science and Medicine* 12, no. 3 (2013): 467-74.

12. H.W. Koh, S.H. Cho, and C.Y. Kim, "Comparison of the Effects of Hollowing and Bracing Exercises on Cross-sectional Areas of Abdominal Muscles in Middle-aged Women," *Journal of Physical Therapy Science* 26, no. 2 (2014): 295-99, doi:10.1589/jpts.26.295.

13. Add this as reference #13: G.J. Dohrmann and N. Mansour, "Long-Term Results of Various Operations for Lumber Disc Herniation: Analysis of Over 39,000 Patients," *Med Princ Pract* 24 (2015): 285-90, doi:10.1159/000375499

Index

Note: The italicized *f* and *t* following page numbers refer to figures and tables, respectively.

About the Author

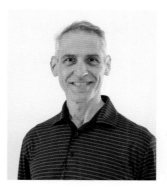

Brian Richey is a personal trainer, educator, and industry leader in the fields of medical exercise and corrective exercise. His unique approach to managing clients' medical conditions through exercise has helped thousands move better, stand taller, and exercise without pain.

Brian earned his BS in kinesiology and exercise science from the University of Hawaii. He has multiple certifications from the American Academy of Health, Fitness, and Rehabilitation Professionals: Medical Exercise Program Director, Medical Exercise Specialist, and Post Rehab Conditioning Specialist. He is a faculty educator and master instructor with Balanced Body.

Brian brings his knowledge in medical exercise, corrective exercise, and integrated movement to the masses through lectures and workshops, both in person and online. He is based in Washington, D.C., where he proudly owns and operates Fit 4 Life DC.

Learn more about Brian Richey at www.BrianRichey.com.

You read the book—now complete the companion CE exam to earn continuing education credit!

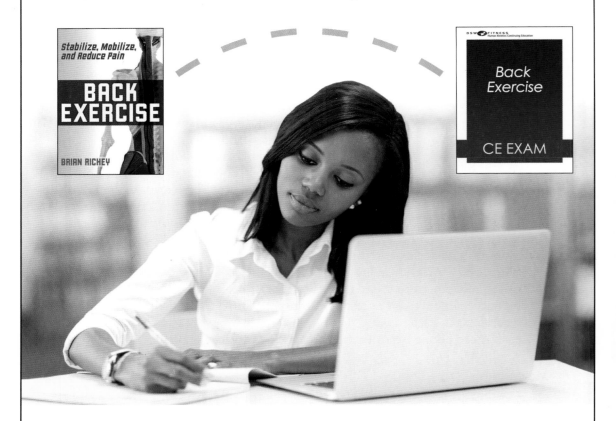

Find and purchase the companion CE exam here:
US.HumanKinetics.com/collections/CE-Exam
Canada.HumanKinetics.com/collections/CE-Exam

50% off the companion CE exam with this code

BE2021

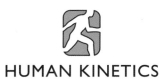

HUMAN KINETICS